# THE WAY OF
# THE SUPERIOR DENTIST

Connecting with Patients, Creating Abundance, and Cultivating your Passion

## ADRIAN WILKINS

Copyright © 2013 Adrian Wilkins
All rights reserved.

ISBN: 1492298956
ISBN 13: 9781492298953

Library of Congress Control Number: 2013916153
CreateSpace Independent Publishing Platform
North Charleston, South Carolina

# CONTENTS

| | |
|---|---|
| Acknowledgments | vii |
| Introduction | ix |
| Part 1: Partner with Everyone | 1 |
| Chapter 1: The Dream | 2 |
|     Burnout | 3 |
|     The Problem | 5 |
|     The Busy Pattern | 6 |
|     Getting off the Merry-Go-Round | 9 |
|     Comprehensive Care Is Not for Everyone | 10 |
|     The General Practice | 11 |
|     Communication or Manipulation? | 12 |
|     Compliance vs. Commitment | 13 |
|     Pushing Patients | 15 |
|     Partner with Everyone, Push No One | 18 |
|     Rapport vs. Relationship | 20 |
| Chapter 2: Intangible Secrets of Success | 24 |
|     Being Present | 26 |
|         Going Deeper | 32 |
|     Appreciation | 35 |
|         Going Deeper | 40 |
|     Hope | 42 |
|         Going Deeper | 47 |
|     Listen, Listen, Listen | 49 |
|         Going Deeper | 54 |
|     About the Intangibles | 56 |

| | |
|---|---|
| Chapter 3: Concepts for Relationship-Centered Dentistry | 58 |
| Why Not Decide for the Patient? | 60 |
| Co-Diagnosis vs. Presenting or Selling | 61 |
| Awareness vs. "You Need" | 63 |
| The Curse of Knowledge | 66 |
| Fear of Scaring the Patient | 68 |
| Trust | 69 |
| The Ostrich | 71 |
| Educating Patients | 73 |
|     Expectations | 74 |
|     Control | 75 |
|     Should vs. Want | 78 |
| Cost and Trust | 78 |
| Speak in Layman's Terms | 81 |
| Analogies, Metaphors, and Similes | 85 |
|     Going Deeper | 87 |
| Identify the Patient's Objectives | 88 |
| Patient Anxiety | 91 |
| Agenda | 95 |
| Commitment | 99 |
| Needs vs. Wants | 101 |
| Paint the Vision | 101 |
| Reinforce Treatment Decisions | 104 |
| Chapter 4: Caretaking and Money | 107 |
| Caretaking vs. Compassion | 107 |
|     Going Deeper | 118 |
| Money | 120 |
|     Dentistry vs. General Medicine | 122 |
|     Strategies for Dealing with Money | 124 |
|     Setting Fees | 124 |
|     Be Real | 125 |
| Going Forward | 127 |
|     Going Deeper | 128 |

| | |
|---|---:|
| Part 2: A Step-by-Step Guide | 131 |
| Chapter 5: Components of Relationship-Centered Dentistry | 132 |
|     Classic Dental Practices | 133 |
|     Relationship-Centered Practice | 133 |
|     Setting the Table | 135 |
|     Consult Room | 135 |
|     Preparation for an Emotional Exam, Clinical Exam, or Review of Findings | 138 |
|     Step 1: Intention | 138 |
|     Step 2: Recording | 139 |
|     Step 3: Break the Ice | 139 |
|     Step 4: Frame the Appointment | 140 |
|     The Comprehensive Exam | 141 |
|         The Emotional Exam | 141 |
|         Clinical Exam | 148 |
|     Co-Discovery | 150 |
|     Photography | 155 |
|     Taking the Photographs | 157 |
|     Photography Equipment | 159 |
|     The Review of Findings Appointment | 160 |
|     Goals and Objectives | 163 |
|     The Tour | 166 |
|     Next Steps | 170 |
|     Periodic and Emergency Exams | 173 |
|         Periodic Exam/Hygiene Check | 173 |
|         Emergency Exam | 175 |
|         Establishing Value for the Comprehensive Exam | 177 |
| Chapter 6: Additional Tools | 179 |
|     Meeting Patients Where They Are | 179 |
|     CAPS Model | 180 |
|         Dominant, Formal—Controller | 182 |
|         Easygoing, Formal—Analyzer | 183 |
|         Dominant, Informal—Promoter | 184 |

| | |
|---|---:|
| Easygoing, Informal—Supporter | 185 |
| How to Use Personality Information | 187 |
| Conclusion | 191 |
| Appendix 1: Hygiene Check, Periodic Exam, and Emergency Exam  Handout | 193 |
| Comprehensive Examinations | 194 |
| Review of Findings Appointment: About Your Next Visit | 196 |
| Appendix 2: Photography Guide | 199 |
| Photography Guide | 201 |
| Appendix 3: Image Used in Picture Exercise | 211 |
| Bibliography | 213 |

## ACKNOWLEDGMENTS

Any major endeavor requires a team to get it done, and I'd like to thank the many people in my life who directly and indirectly supported this effort. Specifically I'd like to thank Dr. Frank Spear, whose pioneering work in dental education for comprehensive care dentistry has been a positive influence on my work over the last fifteen years. In addition, I'd like to thank Ratti Handa, DMD, and Linda Mello, RDH, my two partners in business and friendship. Thank you not just for your technical knowledge but also for your encouragement and the spirit of discovery you helped foster. I would also like to give a special thank you to my editor and friend Jamie Thurber. Jamie was invaluable in getting my words to say what I wanted them to say. But more than that, he was a persistent yet patient force in making this book a reality. Finally, I'd like to thank my partner and wife, Lysa Wilkins, for reminding me of and teaching me joy.

## INTRODUCTION

*Find a job you love and you will
never work a day in your life.*

—CONFUCIUS

"Why did you become a dentist?"

When I meet a new dentist who is interested in my consulting services, this question is always one of the first I ask. The answers vary, of course, depending on who the dentist is and his or her unique personal story. However, even with all the differences, there are some common themes.

At one level or another, most of the doctors I meet want to help people. They also want a profession that affords them a better-than-average income, is challenging, and provides a valuable service to the world.

The obvious follow-up questions are: "How is it going? Are you helping people? Are you making as much money as you had hoped? Are you challenged by the kind of dentistry you are performing? Is dentistry providing the fulfillment you were looking for?" Sometimes the answers are yes, sometimes no, and most often they are somewhere in between. Most of the dentists I meet are really looking to take that next step in their practices; what that step is, however, may not always be clear to them.

There are usually certain common steps dentists seeking to improve their practice have already taken. In addition to the extensive training received in dental school, most continue to sharpen their skills by taking hundreds of hours of continuing education each year. This education often includes complicated prosthodontic training, implant surgery, endodontic training, occlusion training, sedation dentistry, and other specialized instruction. It is not unusual for a dentist to spend tens of thousands of dollars each year on some form of advanced education. But for many, the clinical training does not necessarily mean they will have the opportunity to practice what they have learned. To reconstruct a full mouth or even perform quadrant dentistry, one needs patients who require that kind of work, can afford it, see the value of it, and want it.

Practicing the way you always dreamed is possible! I've lived it with the dentists I support—a complete transformation to the type of practice they have always wanted. To get there, what I'm suggesting is a relationship-centered approach to comprehensive-care dentistry that allows practitioners to provide optimal, whole-mouth care suited for each patient's needs.

This book offers a sound philosophical (part 1) and practical (part 2) foundation for the dentist who wants to perform comprehensive-care dentistry centered on building relationships with patients versus driving them away. The premise is simple: *partner with everyone, push no one.* It's a method any dentist can learn and master. With this approach, you will foster positive relationships with patients who accept treatment. And just as importantly, you'll build strong relationships with patients who do not.

This is more than ideas. It is a step-by-step guide on how to implement the system I will be describing. The philosophical concepts are included right alongside what equipment, systems, and language to use to achieve outstanding results. Part 1 will help you create powerful relationships with patients—a key to successful comprehensive care. Part 2 will provide the practical information about how to create a structure in your practice to operate in this way.

Of note: many dental practices attempt to work within the constraints of dental insurance. This book is not geared toward those who are committed to that approach. On the other hand, it is appropriate for dentists who have worked in that model and are not satisfied with their earning potential or the level of care they are able to offer.

Let me tell you a little about me. I am not a dentist. My background is as a coach and dental practice management consultant. I have not lived your experience, yet at the same time, that has allowed me to step back and see the forest for the trees. Over the past fifteen years, I have had the privilege of working directly with hundreds of dentists—some very successful and some striving to be more successful. I have been fortunate to learn from each and every one of them.

During this time, I have helped new dentists who are becoming established in their practices, dentists going into partnerships, and dentists transitioning at the end of their careers. What we will explore in this book has been refined over thousands of hours with pedodontists, endodontists, periodontists, prosthodontists, oral surgeons, and orthodontists, as well as directly and indirectly with over a thousand general dentists. My coaching and consulting practice includes helping dentists with branding, strategy, operational best practices, and patient communication.

In addition to coaching and consulting to individual doctors and offices, a large part of my practice consists of teaching in the form of lectures and workshops for dentists and teams, particularly in the area of patient communication. I practice daily what I put forth to you here in the hopes of helping dentists to once again love what they do.

You deserve to improve your practice, and you can. With a methodology that makes sense and the specific steps to enact it, you will be able to focus on building your practice through successful relationships with your patients. By incorporating the suggestions in this book into your daily efforts, you will also be well on your way to practicing in the manner many dentists tell me they have always dreamed possible and well on your way to living a happy, healthy, fulfilled life.

# PART 1:

# Partner with Everyone

## CHAPTER 1

# The Dream

*Never continue in a job you don't enjoy. If you're happy in what you're doing, you'll like yourself, you'll have inner peace. And if you have that, along with physical health, you will have had more success than you could possibly have imagined.*

—JOHNNY CARSON

Imagine going to bed at night looking forward to the next day. Imagine getting up before the alarm clock rings, or at the very least being excited to get out of bed when it does ring and not hitting the snooze button. The thought of going to the office is a welcoming and challenging thought and not a stressful one. You arrive with confidence your staff will be there and ready for the new day, your patients are looking forward to seeing you, and you have plenty of profitable work on the schedule.

Instead of rushing from room to room, trying to stay ahead of the amalgams and composites, or worse, not having patients to treat, you are performing the kinds of procedures for which you trained. You have three, four, five, or maybe six patients for the day. These patients are each enthusiastic about receiving comprehensive-care dentistry. Your focus is on delivering quality quadrant and cosmetic dentistry.

Your day consists of productive procedures, fulfilling examinations, and consultations with patients who are grateful to have your services available to them. Most importantly, you work with integrity and walk away from each day feeling energized and alive.

Does this sound like an unrealistic dream to you? For many it does. Is every day going to be like the one described above, completely devoid of any discomfort or stress? Of course not. However, most of the stress in dental offices—and in most jobs, for that matter—is created by us and can be solved by us. Let's take a look at what it is like for many dentists practicing today.

## Burnout

The day starts the previous night. While sliding under the covers, Dr. Smith obsesses about the openings in the next day's schedule and why his front desk manager, Julie, cannot seem to fill them. And when Julie does fill the schedule, patients do not value his time and cancel their appointments. He says to himself, "Tomorrow I am really going to straighten her out." He then remembers that tomorrow morning his first patient is Joe Perkins, and Joe can be tough. He turns over and tries to fall asleep, but it takes a while.

The next morning the alarm goes off, and Dr. Smith slowly comes to life. He gets himself out of bed and prepares for work. Two cups of coffee later, he is ready to face the day. He gets to the office, only to find his assistant is out sick and his second assistant has not prepared all three of the rooms he will be using. Dr. Smith is not sure whether to be upset or relieved that Joe Perkins has no-showed for his appointment. The rest of the day is a blur as Dr. Smith goes from room to room, placing amalgams and composites. He has one crown in the afternoon, but by then, even that does not provide the satisfaction he had hoped for. By the end of the day, Dr. Smith is exhausted. He goes home, has two glasses of wine, and watches the news, where the Dow Jones is down 150 points and he wonders if he will ever retire.

This story is very dramatic and may not completely be representative of your typical day, right? But many dentists struggle daily with not having the kind of office, staff, patients, and treatment they had dreamed of when they became dentists. They make a living but never really accomplish what they had hoped to accomplish. The experience of practicing dentistry is not all they had hoped it would be.

No one starts out hoping to run from room to room performing simple procedures. Nor do they start out wanting a schedule that is unpredictable, with openings throughout the day. So how does it happen? I recently assisted in teaching a course at a local university to third-year dental students. A number of them explained that from day one of their training, they received the message to produce at high rates of speed. In addition, practicing dentists have shared that they started with simple procedures at the beginning of their careers, and it just became comfortable to continue to focus on what they knew well. And their environment—from peers and bosses to their own life experience—taught them that busy and stressed is better. It begins early and stays with most dentists throughout their entire careers. It doesn't have to be this way.

## The Problem

When the answers to any of my, "How's it going?" questions to dentists are less than positive, I often find that the most common tactic used to solve the problem is to advertise and market for new patients. This is done in the hope that if the dentist has more new patients, some will be the type who want the kind of dentistry the doctor wants to provide. By my best estimate, dentists spend over a billion dollars each year advertising for new patients. From phone book advertising to direct mail, television, radio, referral services, and the Internet, the amount of advertising by dentists competing for new patients today is staggering.

With all of the advanced training and all of this advertising, you would expect most dentists to be fulfilling their dreams of performing the best dentistry, giving back to the world, and being compensated consistent with their expertise. Some do achieve those goals, but many do not. Training and an abundance of patients alone are not guarantees. What then is the problem? Why aren't more dentists achieving their personal goals for success?

It is clear that a comfortable patient flow is essential to establishing and maintaining a healthy practice. Without enough patients, an even bigger problem exists because the dentist is likely to be in survival mode. The practitioner is likely to have a scarcity mentality, always worrying that there are not enough patients, and in this frame of mind, the dentist is likely to push away the very patients she wants.

However, it is just as clear that this is *not* the primary reason dentists are not achieving their goals. By any reasonable standard, many of my clients have more patients than they could possibly treat even if only a small percentage chose treatment. Some of my clients and those of other practice consultants have thousands of active patients (active patients being defined as having visited the practice in the last eighteen months) and still are not performing the type or the volume of dentistry they would like.

As you read this book, I would ask you to suspend any beliefs about the need for a high volume of patients to perform the type and amount of dentistry you want to perform. In fact, I can make a strong argument that in many situations, instead of improving the situation, having too many patients contributes to the problem.

If you have been a dentist for a while and have read or listened to even a few dental practice management gurus, you are already familiar with this concept. Because they have seen firsthand the consequences of too many patients, many dental consultants encourage their clients to get off the new patient merry-go-round. It is important to look at this culture of staying busy.

## The Busy Pattern

*I fill my life with a lot of 'busyness' in between jobs. Then I work very hard. Some of it is quite unhealthy. It's compulsive. I don't know what to do about it.*

—HUME CRONYN

Part of the reason we stay so busy is our own discomfort as human beings with doing nothing. If you are not sure what I am talking about, try this. Put this book down for a few minutes. Assuming you are alone, shut off any electronics, including computer, TV, and radio. Then look at your watch and sit quietly for five minutes. During that time, do not speak, and try your best to just be there without thinking or doing. This means sitting quietly without planning for the future or thinking about the past. This means just sitting without having any thoughts in your mind at all. Avoid even the thought that you will not have any thoughts! After you are finished, turn to the next page. All right, begin now…

How did you do? If you actually suspended all thought for those five minutes, congratulations; you are, by almost all spiritual standards, enlightened. If you found it difficult to sit quietly without thinking, don't feel bad; you are like many of us. And if you found a reason not to do it at all, you are probably in the majority.

Most of us find it very difficult to do nothing. Many people describe a sense of anxiety when doing nothing. We possess a strong internal emotional pull to think and do. Human beings are for the most part thinking and doing machines. Left alone, most people will immediately start to do something or at least start to think. It's interesting since we call ourselves "human beings," not "human doers."

It is no surprise that our natural tendency is to try to fill the time with something to do. Put that tendency together with the conventional dental wisdom of working, being busy every moment, and a new dentist's need to earn income for survival, and it is easy to see why many dentists emphasize filling the schedule.

Unfortunately, this approach has some negative consequences. Imagine the new dentist just starting out. She[1] typically has just finished eight years or more of training and is eager to put her talents to use. Unless she is very fortunate, she is likely saddled with some pretty hefty student loans and needs to begin earning money quickly.

Many dentists start out as associates in someone else's practice. The owner dentist often gives the new associate the children and less-complicated cases. Even if the owner does not filter the patients sent to the new dentist, the staff tends to direct the more-complicated cases to the owner.

---

1 Since today the number of women entering dentistry is on the rise and it is cumbersome to keep stating "he or she," for purposes of simplicity, I will refer to the dentist as she in the first half of the book and he in the second half.

In the early stages of being an associate, there are some important factors in play. The associate, for the reasons discussed above, needs money. In addition, the associate has not yet become proficient at treating complicated cases. Starting out, most new associates do not receive as many patients as they perceive they need. The result is that new dentists, who probably have a greater need for income starting out their careers than the dentists who are well established in life, find themselves needing treatment in their chairs and needing it now.

The new dentist might decide that rather than sit around for an hour, it may be better to do that prophy for Mrs. Jones. Or perhaps a patient comes in needing quite a bit of restorative work, but the dentist has open time and a desire to make money immediately, so she places a small amalgam instead, right on the spot. The urgency to be busy encourages the dentist to schedule treatment as quickly as possible to satisfy her own needs.

There is another factor to consider, and that is patients are meeting the young new associate for the first time. The new associate is likely between twenty-six and twenty-eight years of age and typically does not possess the same presence as an experienced dentist. The young associate may be a little less confident in suggesting comprehensive care, and the patient may be a little less confident in the young dentist. For this reason, the patient and the dentist may both be more comfortable starting out with smaller treatments.

Let's take a closer look at this situation. The new dentist fills the schedule with small treatments. She needs more treatments because she needs the revenue, and pretty soon the schedule starts to fill up. The result is smaller gaps in the schedule, leaving room for more small treatments but not the large treatments that ultimately both patient and practitioner would prefer. This new dentist finds herself in a perfect storm of new patients, a strong need for income, and a greater comfort level with smaller procedures, which leads to the dentist performing smaller and smaller treatments and establishing a pattern that is difficult to change.

This situation snowballs, and pretty soon the new dentist finds herself seeing ten to twenty patients a day in her main column and others in hygiene. Running from one patient to another, these dentists are almost certain to continue on the same track. Most are not fully conscious of how they got to where they are. The ones who are aware may have decided that once they are busy they will change, but they find it difficult to get off the merry-go-round.

Once the new associate is busy, even if the dentist has the wisdom to recognize the problem, it becomes very difficult to change the established pattern. In this situation, I typically see a dentist who has many patients performing small procedures for a number of years and who is beginning to experience burnout. The profile of this dentist is of someone who wants to practice better, more-comprehensive dentistry and is tired of drilling and filling all day but needs the money for survival and does not know how to change the pattern. Further, the very powerful emotional tendency most of us have to want to be busy and avoid sitting still dramatically raises the level of difficulty to make this important change to a better way of practicing dentistry.

## Getting off the Merry-Go-Round

*When you're on a merry-go-round, you miss a lot of the scenery.*

—NEIL DIAMOND

The recognition of the dangers of too many patients explains why some practice consultants and dentists advocate a comprehensive care–only style of practice. I believe their intention is positive in that they want to provide great care for the patient and a fulfilling experience for the dentist. However, some of these approaches advocate what can be described as an either-or approach.

Either the patient is interested in accepting optimal treatment or the dentist should refuse to treat the patient any other way.

Advocates of this approach suggest that performing anything less than optimal care is a form of *supervised neglect*. Much of the emphasis is on attracting the right type of patients and then educating and convincing patients why they should choose comprehensive care.

The desire to educate patients and make it possible for them to get the best care is admirable. Clearly, patients who need, want, and can afford the best dental care benefit from this method. And the dentist is able to practice the way she strives to practice. So what's the problem?

## Comprehensive Care Is Not for Everyone

The problem is that not everyone can afford or values comprehensive care. For those of us involved in dentistry, that can be hard to hear. We want to believe that if we do a good job of communicating this approach, the patient will accept it. It's even possible to convince oneself that if someone really values the care, then there is always a way to manage the money issues.

However, although many of these things are true, many patients simply will never choose comprehensive care regardless of what we do. Worse, others will get care because of what one can only describe as manipulation, and ultimately they will resent it.

The reality is that many patients are great candidates for comprehensive care, and some are not. The problem begins when we try to force the latter into the former category.

There are dentists who have found a way to avoid the problem. If you are a prosthodontist and your brand is clear, you only treat complicated cases. And assuming you have a sufficient number of referring dentists who prequalify your potential patients, you are in great shape. The patients coming to you are probably the right patients, and even if a patient decides not to accept treatment, he at least understands why he is in your chair in the first place. If you do a reasonable job of presenting to patients their needs and options and you have a reasonable number of good candidates being referred, you should be in good shape.

## The General Practice

However, most dentists and some specialists are in a different position. If they are fortunate, they have a steady flow of patients with needs varying from basic maintenance to complicated advanced treatment. Some of these patients need and want comprehensive-care dentistry. If you partner with these patients in the manner described in this book, you will have an excellent level of success.

On the other hand, the majority of patients the general dentist's office will encounter are not immediately prepared for and do not want comprehensive-care dentistry. It may be that they are just beginning to understand they have significant needs. Or they may not value the type of dentistry we have been talking about. Or they may simply not be able to afford the kind of work that is likely in their best interests.

This is where the dilemma for the general dentist begins. Some advocates of comprehensive-care dentistry suggest encouraging all patients to choose their method. Further, many of them propose methods of communication that, in effect, pressure the patient to accept the type of treatment they feel is in the patient's best interests.

Most of these proponents of comprehensive-care dentistry really do have the patient's best interests at the heart of their philosophy. My sense is they feel strongly that many patients do not understand how important it is to treat the whole mouth as opposed to individual teeth. Unfortunately, in the effort to get this message across to patients and other dentists, this approach can take on the quality of a crusade for better dentistry.

## Communication or Manipulation?

*A life lived with integrity - even if it lacks the trappings of fame and fortune is a shining star in whose light others may follow in the years to come.*

—DENIS WAITLEY

As the dentist examines and forms a treatment plan, she encounters patients who either do not understand or understand and do not want the care being recommended. These dentists in turn work harder and harder on their communication skills. They offer financing methods to make it easier for the patient to afford treatment, and they learn sales techniques for overcoming objections.

I will never forget one of my earliest memories of one of these sales techniques. I was in my early twenties, and I walked into a large retail store. At the front of the store stood a temporary concession stand with a salesman selling relatively inexpensive watches. As I walked by the table of watches, one of them caught my eye. Until this point in my life, I had never worn a watch and was curious. I wanted to look at a few and consider the idea of wearing one. I was at the stage of exploration and understanding and not even close to being ready to buy one.

The salesman had me try on a few watches and finally asked me if I would like to buy the one I had been looking at. I told him I would like to *think* about it. He then asked me if I thought the watch looked good on me. I answered yes. He asked me if I thought it was a fair price, and I said yes. He then asked me if I thought Waltham watches were good watches. And I answered that I guessed they were. He then said to me, "Now that you have *thought* about it, would you like to buy the watch?"

It was clever, and though I didn't buy it, for a twenty-year-old it was difficult to say no. But more importantly, it was the first time I really thought about sales in a negative way. I felt very pressured and manipulated. If you try, I am sure you can think of many examples or versions of similar "overcome the objections" sales techniques I am talking about.

I suppose if one's goal is to sell a few watches to people you will never see again, the technique above could be effective. However, if the goal is to partner with patients and foster long-term relationships, this would not be the method I would recommend.

## Compliance vs. Commitment

*Choose your love, Love your choice.*

—THOMAS S. MONSON

Most of us would characterize manipulation as a negative attribute. Then why do some dentists resort to manipulation? The truth is that pressure and manipulation sometimes work, at least in the short term. I am sure the watch salesman sold quite a few watches that day. You may, through clever techniques, get patients to accept treatment they otherwise would not choose. And for many, the justification is that patients end up getting the treatment they need, and the dentist gets to perform and reap the rewards of performing the type of treatment she enjoys.

Unfortunately, even putting aside ethical considerations, this type of case presentation technique has major drawbacks. If the dentist is successful in convincing the patient to accept treatment over objections, at some fundamental level the patient is not fully committed to treatment. These are the patients who do it because the dentist wants them to. Maybe they go forward because they do not want to disappoint the dentist. Maybe they think they "should." Maybe they just do not know how to say no.

Whatever their reason, they have some reservations; otherwise there would be no objection to overcome. Many of these are the patients who cancel or do not keep their scheduled appointments. Or sometimes this is the patient who goes forward with treatment and then is unhappy with some aspect of the result. These are often the patients who do not pay their bills because they resent having been coerced into treatment. Not paying can be a more common way of expressing dissatisfaction than many realize.

If they do show for their appointments, do not complain, and pay their bills, they often tell their friends how they just spent twenty-five thousand dollars at the dentist and compare you to something like paying the IRS: something they have to but did not want to do. In this scenario, too many patients are dissatisfied, and the consequences to that specific relationship and the reputation created in the community are not what most of us would consciously choose.

What concerns me is that this is the best-case scenario. In this situation, the patient completes the treatment but is not really on board. Even worse is the patient we try to convince who does not accept. How does he feel? How does he behave? What does he go outside and tell other potential patients about your practice?

I have spoken to many patients who have been to offices where the approach is one of convincing patients to accept treatment they did not want or could not afford. Do these patients turn to the dentist and tell her they are unhappy at what they perceive as pressure? In a few cases, they do. This is the patient who asks you if he is "putting your kids through college." Or he tells you bluntly that he does not want to hear about comprehensive-care dentistry.

However, more often than not, they say nothing. That's right, nothing. They may continue to come in for cleanings and beg or insist the hygienist not call you into the room. But more often, they vote with their feet. They say, "Thank you, Doctor Jones," and then they go home and never come back. They call their insurance companies or look on the Internet and find another dentist. And if this is all they did, it would be bad enough, but it isn't. They tell person after person their dental version of my watch story. The impact does not take long to feel. Before you know it, hundreds of people have told thousands of patients to stay away from your practice.

*The most valuable asset any of us have is our reputation, and nothing destroys our reputation faster than negative word of mouth.*

Compliant patients, while they appear beneficial in the short term, are not the long-term answer. And if what they say about you does harm to your reputation, they may well be a long-term death-of-practice sentence.

## Pushing Patients

I have been involved in quite a number of practice transitions, from that of retiring dentists to relatively young practitioners. One of the common scenarios is of the very likeable, low-key, low-pressure dentist selling her practice. Usually this dentist is someone who saw her patients for cleanings, never did a comprehensive exam, kept fees relatively low, and only did crown and bridge work on patients who were in obvious and serious need.

A description of this type of dentist might look something like, "She's a nice lady and doesn't push all this fancy stuff." This style of dentist attracts a large number of patients over the years. When a tooth has decay, she places an amalgam; when the amalgam fails, she places a larger one. Finally she may place a crown, but often she or the patient opts for an extraction. From the patients' perspective, this is the natural progression, and perhaps, eventually, the patients will wear dentures like their parents. This is the natural order of things, and the dentist is rarely blamed.

Then the new dentist arrives, and at first things are great. I have seen many dentists take over and start pushing comprehensive care, and at first the results are astounding. Though they push the patients, they double (or more) the revenues of the selling doctor in the first year. But sometimes right away, and sometimes a little further into the transition, the dentist states that she has lost some patients. At first the loss is attributed to the doctor being new or maybe that these are the bad patients who she does not mind losing.

As time goes on, more patients are lost, but business continues to be pretty good because there is just so much dentistry that needs to be done when following a dentist who did not believe in comprehensive care. Finally, usually a year or two later, the buyer starts to get concerned that she does not have enough patients. Before your eyes, you can watch this type of practice go from feast to famine, and it is amazing how it does not take long to erode a once-healthy patient base.

This problem of losing patients is often compounded by the fact that the retiring dentist, by her practice style, attracted many patients who were more comfortable going to a dentist who tended to suggest minimal treatment plans. If the patients who do not yet have a long-term relationship with the new dentist are then told they need comprehensive care, they feel further pressured by these methods. The point is that there is a direct correlation between pressuring patients about treatment and a lack of patients. I have watched this process occur many times, and it is clear to me that in the process of advocating comprehensive-care dentistry, it is very important to do it in such a way that we do not alienate patients.

The typical general practice patient base is made up of different types of patients. Some understand the value, have the resources, and are open to the concept of comprehensive-care dentistry. Others do not understand but are easily educated, and once that is accomplished, they are generally on board. Still others understand or are open to learning but do not have the resources. Finally there are patients who for various reasons do not value better dentistry, and education is not the issue.

One way of dealing with this mix of patients is to have the owner act as a specialist within the general practice. You see this with an experienced owner and a younger associate. Usually the owner has a large patient base and cannot give all of her patients the time she would like to give them. Further, as her career has evolved, there is an interest in performing more of the complex procedures for which she has trained. The recognition that not all of the patients need or want this type of care causes the owner to look for someone to treat patients requiring less dentistry.

At first glance, this seems to be a reasonable approach. It certainly works better than trying to put a square peg into a round hole by pushing comprehensive-care dentistry on patients who are not a good fit. It also provides services to those patients who have not bought into or are unable to afford comprehensive-care dentistry. And it has the added benefit of giving the owner time to spend with the candidates who are right for more comprehensive care. In comparing it to the alternatives of providing minimal care to everyone or pushing everyone toward comprehensive care, it is definitely a better option.

However, this approach also has its drawbacks. It is very difficult to get a qualified associate who is willing to perform basic dentistry without being allowed to do more complicated cases. In addition, there are problems in terms of diagnosing and referring to the senior dentist. Patients also tend to be put off when they are shuffled to a different dentist.

ADRIAN WILKINS

## Partner with Everyone, Push No One

I propose a different approach. Partner with everyone without pressuring anyone. This way all of your patients are offered comprehensive care. Some will do it and some will not, but almost everyone will stay.

Makes sense, right? So why do most dentists not do it this way? It seems so obvious, and I have seen it work. So why write a book about something that most would describe as common sense?

As with most things, the concept is simple but the execution is not. There are a number of factors that need to be addressed for this approach to work. They include concrete issues, such as the amount of time spent with patients, maintaining productivity, and the established routines of the doctor. Then there are some less-tangible and typically unconscious factors, such as patient expectations, doctor beliefs, and staff beliefs that operate in the background but need to be recognized and addressed.

However, the results when this concept is applied can be described as nothing short of astounding. I have personally witnessed doctors take their practices to new heights by embracing and applying the principles described in this book.

In one situation, a dentist purchased a practice from a retiring dentist with approximately three hundred active patients and a very poor reputation who was collecting approximately thirty thousand dollars per month. By applying the principles in this book, she turned the business into a full-time practice, collecting ninety thousand dollars per month with virtually no external marketing in a little less than nine months! During that time, the patient base stayed approximately the same.

At the end of a year, the practice was up to $110,000 per month in collections, the schedule was booked out two months, plans for external marketing were put on hold, and the patient loyalty in the practice was as strong as I have ever seen. Clearly this doctor is exceptional, and the credit for her success is not all the result of applying the principles in this book. However, she would tell you that her success in no small part was significantly impacted by learning how to effectively communicate comprehensive care to a patient base that had lost trust with the prior owner.

In another case, I witnessed a dentist with an established practice apply these principles and achieve equally remarkable results. This dentist had spent years marketing heavily to try to increase his business. The marketing was successful in that he had grown the business to in excess of $120,000 per month, but the type of patient was not what he wanted, the cost of advertising was significantly eroding his profits, and his personal satisfaction and that of his staff was less than desired. He did plan treatment for comprehensive-care dentistry, and some accepted but many did not. The ones who did often struggled around finances, and the relationship between the practice and the patient at times was adversarial.

Unlike the first dentist, he did not have a natural talent for patient communication and was concerned with whether he would be able to apply the concepts in this book. With several months of study and practice, he was able to implement much of what has been described here.

In less than six months, his practice grew another 10 percent. But more importantly, his advertising costs dropped dramatically, his relationship with his patients improved, and most importantly, his personal experience of practicing went from one of constant stress to one of really enjoying the practice of dentistry.

These are just two of the many dentists who have applied these principles and improved their practices and their lives. Will you achieve these same results? That depends on where you start from, how naturally talented you are, and how hard you work at this. However, if you bring genuine effort to the process, you will improve your practice dramatically.

ADRIAN WILKINS

## Rapport vs. Relationship

*I love you, and because I love you, I would sooner have you hate me for telling you the truth than adore me for telling you lies.*

—PIETRO ARETINO

Since this book is about relationship-centered dentistry, it may be helpful if we begin to define relationship the way we intend it in this book. If you ask the average dentist, she will probably tell you she has an excellent relationship with her patients. She might tell you how much her patients like her and enjoy her company. She might be one of those dentists with a knack for remembering names and personal information about patients and their families, such as where they live, where they go to school, who they know, and what they do with their spare time. Further, when the patient comes in, the doctor and patient might find themselves talking through the whole appointment in a friendly manner, with smiles and positive body language. It is easy to see how this dentist would conclude she has excellent relationships with her patients. However, I would say to you that this dentist has excellent rapport with her patients and may, but probably does not, have excellent relationships with them.

Let's look at the difference between rapport and relationship. With great rapport, we tend to like and be liked by the other person. We seem to have a lot in common or have an interest in the same things. Great rapport is what we often feel when we meet someone at a party or gathering and right away we like him or her. It can be a staff member patients rave about or really like or even love. Great rapport is almost always the first step to create a powerful relationship with a patient, but in and of itself, great rapport is not enough.

If you are wondering whether having great rapport equals having a great relationship, I would suggest trying on these two statements and asking yourself which one feels right: "I have great rapport with my husband" or "I have a great relationship with my husband." When you look at it this way, it is obvious that with the people who are most important to us, we want more than rapport. We want something deeper. We want a powerful relationship.

So what makes a great relationship? What takes us further and deeper than rapport? It is difficult to describe precisely, but great relationships generally include the following:

- *Deep Listening.* This means I listen, you listen, and we both learn.

- *Spontaneity.* Great relationships include the niceties and perfunctory comments like, "How are you today?" but they also include the possibility of something completely unexpected! For this reason, real relationships are exciting.

- *Risking.* Can you remember back to the early stages of an important courtship? Maybe you talked until all hours of the morning, sharing intimate details about each other's lives, not knowing for sure how the other person would respond. You took risks with each other, and the relationship felt really alive. For many people, as time went on, some of that excitement and risking got replaced by dealing with the issues of daily life, from who will feed the dog to who will take out the trash. But in the midst of these day-to-day issues, there are moments where we go deeper with each other and touch that early stage of sharing and risking.

- *Challenge.* In a real relationship, we are willing to challenge each other. The more I care about you, the more I am willing to say something to you that may be difficult for you to hear. I care more about you achieving your goals than whether you like me. There is probably no place where this is truer than with our children.

- ❖ *Openness.* In a real relationship, we are open about our agendas. If there is something we want from the other person, we do not hide it but rather tell him or her. Real relationships are valued and cannot be replaced easily. In fact, most of us would agree that a true friend is not easy to find.

This book is about creating real relationships with your patients—relationships that go way beyond rapport. In fact, it's possible that you will learn and know some of your patients' deepest hopes and fears about their dental health and never know their favorite restaurants. I have seen countless dentists who were surprised and disappointed that a patient with whom they had great rapport left their practice because of price, because of a billing error, or because the dentist no longer participated in the patient's dental insurance. And although the same thing can happen when you are in relationship with your patients, it is much less likely. I have seen very successful fee-for-service practices built on the concept of having real relationships with their patients.

As stated above, a good friendship is rare. When you have a powerful relationship with your patients, they will have very powerful reasons to stay with you through the difficult challenges that often face the dentist-patient relationship. In the next chapter, we will explore some of the intangible secrets of success that help to build the kinds of relationships we have been talking about.

## Summary of Key Points

- ❖ *Find a job you love.* Create the practice of your dreams rather than hoping it will find you.

- ❖ *Comprehensive care is not for everyone.* Some patients are candidates, and some are not.

- *Communication or manipulation?* Avoid being seduced by the desire to overcome objections.

- *Commitment instead of compliance.* Why patients say yes is more important than whether they say yes.

- *Partner with everyone and push no one.* Utilize an approach that is valued as much by the patients who do not go forward with treatment as those who do.

- *Rapport vs. Relationship.* Go beyond being nice, and create a powerful partnership that helps your patients achieve optimal health.

> **Note:** Most dental offices are familiar with Clinical, Periodic, and Emergency Exams. We will be talking about two other types of exams in this book: an Emotional Exam and a Review of Findings Appointment. The Emotional Exam is an appointment to learn about the patient before you start working on him clinically. Or another way of saying it, it's a way to learn about the person behind the teeth. The Review of Findings appointment occurs after the Clinical Exam, either the same day or on a separate appointment, during which time we explore what was learned during the Clinical Exam. We'll describe both of these types of exams and the overall structure of the process later in the book.

# CHAPTER 2

# Intangible Secrets of Success

*In essence, if we want to direct our lives, we must take control of our consistent actions. It's not what we do once in a while that shapes our lives, but what we do consistently.*

—TONY ROBBINS

Many books have been written about the key principles of relating to and influencing others. I have read many books about communication and have studied hundreds of principles, many of which I have found to be useful in relating to the people around me.

But there are certain things we learn in our lives that we understand from more than a theoretical place within ourselves; we understand these things from a place of experience and true knowing—a place where no matter how much we are challenged, there is confidence in the truth of what we believe.

For me, what I am preparing to explain has that kind of truth. Over the years, I have had significant experience in selling, coaching, and communicating with acquaintances and clients and have become clear about some of the critical elements that work to create successful relationships. These are things found to be at the core of virtually all of the interactions that created a positive result for both the other person and for me. These truths or intangible factors are critical to this method. If you concentrate on mastering them, it will go a long way toward building effective relationships with your patients.

These intangible factors require a different type of learning that is not as concrete as other forms of acquiring knowledge. For example, discussing how much time to allot for a comprehensive exam is pretty straightforward compared to exploring the issue of patient trust.

The reality, though, is that becoming competent in the intangible areas of working with patients makes a huge difference to the success of a dentist. I have worked with many technically exceptional dentists who could not fill up their schedules with fulfilling work simply because of their inability to foster healthy relationships with their patients. In essence, these are the foundational building blocks to successfully partnering with your patient and really, to partnering with people in your life: being present, appreciation, hope, and listening (see figure 1).

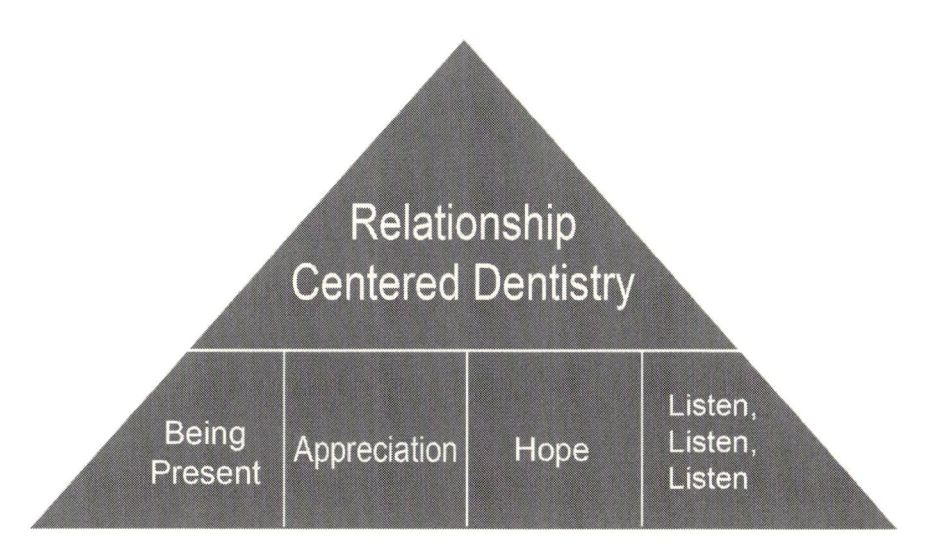

Figure 1: The intangibles are the foundation for Relationship Centered Dentistry.

## Being Present

*Do not dwell in the past, do not dream of the future, concentrate the mind on the present moment.*

—BUDDHA

In the world of partnering and working with patients, when distilled to its purest element, the most basic and most important intangible is the ability of the dentist to be present. Being present means being right here, right now, without the fears of tomorrow and the regrets of the past distracting us. For our purposes, we will talk about being present to mean having passion and connecting with our true selves and in turn, connecting with the patient. This ability to connect with ourselves and others is truly priceless. Most of us spend our lives trying to connect with the ones closest to us at the deepest level. Whether that connection is between husband and wife, parent and child, or friends, the desire to connect and the experience of connection is powerful. People who are successful in connecting with themselves and with others, and who are able to enroll others in their vision, will find the world opening up to them.

But what does this being present look like?

I have a colleague who describes a moment with his twelve-year-old son. His son, a gymnast, had just finished a high-level meet in Las Vegas, one that he'd prepared to compete in for many months. He'd fallen on the rings and the pommel horse, and he'd taken several extra steps on the floor routine.

"He had a tough meet," my colleague said, "and we stood off to the side, me up above leaning over a railing and he still in his singlet down in the competing area, looking out over the floor with the many parents and friends of the gymnasts on the bleachers behind him. I could see that he was upset, and my heart broke. I felt this strong desire to make it OK for him, to take away that pain. But something held me back from rushing in to fix it, and I felt I was right there with him in that moment.

"It sounds kind of funny, but the people in the stands went into the background, and the sounds of many voices and loudspeakers seemed to dim, and it was just him and me. I asked him, 'How are you doing?' He looked away from me, then back, and I could see his eyes just beginning to water. He said, 'I just feel disappointed in myself because I know I could have done better.' And I could see that disappointment hanging on him, but in a way, I could also see him let go of it a little bit, just because there was space for him to say it. I felt myself hold my breath for a second, unsure of what to say or do, still feeling the pull to fix it. Then I let go of my breath, and I simply said, 'I love you, buddy.' He said, 'I love you, too, Dad.' I felt such a connection to him and to me in that moment, and I could see that he'd be OK—not because of something I'd done but rather because I was able to just be there with him, letting him experience his experience, just witnessing the beautiful process of a human being coming to terms with himself. I'll never forget it."

Very simply, he was present with himself and his son. And in that seemingly simple act, a very powerful moment emerged.

This concept of being present is in and of itself the subject of thousands of spiritual and psychological books. Buddha is quoted as having said, "You shouldn't chase after the past or place expectations on the future. What is past is left behind. The future is as yet unreached. Whatever quality is present you clearly see right there, right there." Christianity talks about being present as being a quality related to the divine. Most religions and philosophies extoll the virtues of being present in the moment.

This is the same energy, or way of being, that helps a patient feel connected to his doctor and inspired to work with that dentist. All of us know dentists whose patients simply do whatever the dentist suggests. Why? The dentists I am talking about generally do not perform the technically best case presentation. It is common for these very successful communicators to say nothing more than, "You need five crowns, two root canals, and an implant," and the patient says "OK." They do not use photos, x-rays, or instructional videos. They simply recommend treatment, and the patient accepts the treatment. If you asked them how they did it, they probably could not tell you. It is a little like a six-year-old who can put a sentence together with the proper syntax without knowing the definition of a verb or a noun or the rules for using them.

Do not interpret what I am saying to suggest that technique is not important. It is very important. I would not write a book about effective communication if I did not think it was important. These very successful communicators generally accomplish many of the objectives found in a successful case presentation. They do it a little like the six-year-old: without knowing they are doing it. But as successful as many of these dentists are, they would be even more successful if they could take their raw talent for communication and fine tune it with better technique. In the end, no matter how you look at case presentation and life, the ability to connect emotionally and passionately is often the difference between success and failure.

We may not always know how to connect ourselves, but we can almost always recognize this ability in others. If you stop and think about famous communicators like Ronald Reagan, John F. Kennedy, or any of the thousands of people throughout history who inspired people to follow them, they all had the ability one way or another to connect with the people they led.

But we do not need to look at historical figures and world leaders to find this quality. All of us have people in our lives with whom we are grateful to have crossed paths. Usually there is an energy surrounding these people that is unmistakable. It is not something specific they say or do that creates that feeling. There is a passion, an intimacy, and an aliveness we just want to be near. This person could be a husband, a wife, a friend, an employee, or a boss.

When we are with them, we have the uncanny feeling that they are treating us like the most important person in the room. They can be rich or they can be poor, but what they all have in common is that we walk away feeling better for having been in their presence.

I once sat in on a meeting with two salespeople. The junior salesperson did almost all of the talking. He was a nice enough guy and did a good job. The senior salesperson said very little, but he had a way about him that left an impression. I noticed it during the meeting, and after the meeting, the client and I were talking about the session, and the client immediately pointed out that he had noticed the same thing. He said something to the effect that the senior salesperson was really great. I estimate this senior salesperson did 5 percent of the talking, yet the client and I could both feel his presence. People with presence have an energy about them that goes deeper than knowledge, words, or body language.

Another way of thinking about being present or connected is to think about moments in your life that were "just right." Maybe you were on vacation or in nature watching a sunset or the moon. You experienced peacefulness and a connection in which the world felt exactly as it was meant to be.

I had such a moment when I first met my wife. I had just been through a tough period when my life had taken a difficult turn, and I found myself in a long period of heaviness. I felt ready to move on and invite a new relationship into my life, and as I sat and meditated, I had a deep sense of peace and a strong feeling I had met the person I would spend the rest of my life with. It was like it had already happened but just not yet in the physical world.

Later on the same day, I took a walk in the mountains near my house. I remember it being a sunny, warm day, with the light illuminating the green up in the hills. I felt at peace, and as I thought about my morning meditation, a woman came into my vision on a path up ahead, riding a chestnut-brown horse. I felt a sense of beauty and knowing and lightness in my body, and I knew in that moment I would meet her and this was the one. It was a perfect, just-right moment for me.

For you, maybe it was your wedding day, or maybe it was watching your child in a school play. It could even be the sense of confidence performing a new procedure and realizing in that moment you were bringing all of your intention and ability to your work, and it became effortless. When describing feeling present, people often will describe a sense of flow or effortlessness. Time passes quickly. If you feel like you are working hard at something and are pushing yourself to do it, you are more than likely not in the flow or fully present with yourself.

Take a few minutes now to reflect on your "just right" moments. I suggest getting a pen and paper and reflecting on one or two special times in your life that felt "just right." Then sit and commit those experiences to writing. Write about exactly what you were doing, where you were, what you experienced, what it felt like emotionally, and what about those moments in time made them so special.

After writing them down, think about what your professional life would be like if you could bring those powerful feelings into your work world. Many people make the mistake of believing these feelings of connection and presence only come to us through luck or just the right circumstances. This is because most of us do not believe we have control over our own experiences. We experience life a little like a small boat on a large ocean, being tossed around by the giant waves. We are grateful when there is a calm moment on the sea but feel we have nothing to do with creating the calm waters. Being present brings these calm waters.

Certainly in our personal and work lives, there are many things that are out of our control. But the people who are the most effective and enjoy life the most are the ones who have learned to have a balance between controlling what they can control and accepting what they cannot. These people often are able to have more choice over how they experience their world than the rest of us do.

This subject of passion, presence, and emotional connection has been the topic of thousands of books, artists, philosophers, and management gurus. It is unrealistic to believe that in a section of this book we can fully teach something that takes many a lifetime to learn and that the vast majority of us never fully master.

But what we can do is introduce you to some of the concepts surrounding presence and emotional connection. Not everyone has the raw talent to be a concert pianist. But virtually all of us can learn enough to play our favorite tunes. There is innate ability as it relates to our communication skills, and there are principles and techniques that can be learned.

And this is really what it's about. Being present with yourself allows you to be present with your patients. During exams, you are able to be there solely with your patients and their needs. There's no worrying about bills or a procedure to come but just what this patient needs right now. Ultimately that will allow you to fully understand the patient's needs and better provide treatment options, which will lead to more patients wanting work done. But mostly it will allow you to better connect with your patients.

In addition, it is important to note that these are the same qualities that impact all of our close relationships. Not only will you become a better communicator and connect with your patients, but perhaps more importantly, you will learn to communicate and connect with yourself and those close to you.

To help you practice, in each of the intangible sections, I include a "Going Deeper" section in which I suggest ways you might bring this intangible further into your life. These are lifetime practices.

## Going Deeper

Here are a few practices that can help you with being present.

1. Daily, it is important to find ways to bring yourself back to now, especially in locations where you are used to following patterns that don't serve you. Hang up Post-it notes in places that disrupt your routine and remind you of coming back to this moment. When you see the Post-it, stop what you're doing, take a deep breath, and think of your Just Right Moment. To keep you noticing them, move the Post-its once a week (or better yet, have your staff move them so you will be surprised).

2. Set aside at least two minutes each day to connect deeply with someone you care about. Speak about matters that are truly important to you. Be vulnerable. As you continue the practice, increase the amount of time by one minute, perhaps each month. Being truly present with another is one of the greatest gifts we can give ourselves.

3. Practice meditation. Can anyone achieve the same calmness, joy, and focus that are often shown by Buddhist monks in the face of great hardships? Many studies say yes, from those conducted by UC Davis to those by Stanford University, in which they studied the effects of meditation on the brain.[2, 3] Their findings suggest that those who meditate are much less likely to be like that small boat being thrown haphazardly onto a big sea. Rather than react, they can choose.

---

2  Smith, *Shamatha Project*
3  Hutcherson, Seppala, & and Gross, *Loving-Kindness Meditation Increases Social Connectedness*, 720-24

4. In terms of dentistry, meditation can help you to be more present with your patients, better able to listen to them rather than to be a passenger on their emotional roller coasters. The basic concept of meditation is to focus and allow thoughts to pass by. It's a little like lying on your back, staring up at the clouds, and watching them glide past. Your thoughts are like those clouds, and you let them come and go but don't grab them. Our minds are like gardens that need tending; without tending, they become overgrown with weeds and become difficult to navigate. Meditation allows us to clear the weeds and create space for the garden to bloom. I highly encourage you to take up a practice. Start small and see how it feels for you. A few techniques are listed below.

   a. Four-four-eight. You can practice this meditation anywhere, in a short period of time. You might use it prior to entering an exam room. First, breathe in for a count of four, and as you do, picture a place in your life that brings you great joy. Then hold your breath for the count of four. Finally, release your breath slowly, on a count of eight, and feel your body release any stress.

   b. Walking Meditation. Allow the simple act of walking to bring you back to the present moment. Take twenty to thirty minutes to walk slowly and deliberately, feeling the support of the earth as your feet come in contact with it. It's best done outdoors but can be done indoors as well. The technique described below is based on a Tibetan practice of Thich Nhat Hanh.[4] In essence, it is about enjoying each step and all that is around you. Choose a length of time that works for you, though twenty to thirty minutes is generally a good starting

---

4 Hanh, *Art of Mindful Living—Walking Meditation*.

point. As you walk, simply notice what is going on around you—the sounds of birds, the sun beaming down on you, the feel of the wind in its travels. With each step, feel gratitude for this earth. Take two to three steps for each in breath and out breath, breathing slowly. To focus your mind, it may help to use a mantra such as the following:

c. *Breathing in, "I have arrived"; Breathing out, "I am home"*
   *Breathing in, "In the here"; Breathing out, "In the now"*
   *Breathing in, "I am solid"; Breathing out, "I am free"*
   *Breathing in, "In the ultimate"; Breathing out, "I dwell"*

To support your practice, you may find it helpful to seek meditation groups in your area. Internet search engines with the words "meditation near {insert location}" can lead you to such groups. Either way, be gentle with yourself because it takes time, and when you first start, it may seem very difficult. Our minds are so full of thoughts we've learned and cultivated that we operate almost like an .mp3 player—push a button and a song plays, almost without our being conscious of it. A person cuts you off on the highway, and you react back with anger. A friend doesn't call you back, and you feel unloved. A co-worker yells, and you react out of fear. Meditation helps you to quiet the reactions, clear the mind, and choose.

## Appreciation

*It is not our purpose to become each other; it is to recognize each other, to learn to see the other and honor him for what he is.*

—HERMANN HESSE

The second intangible is appreciation. By most standards, I am relatively shy and not what someone would describe as charismatic. But I consider myself incredibly fortunate in that, either because of my nature or my life experiences, I really like people. You will notice that I did not say people like me. Some people like me and some do not. However, what I have found to be more important than people liking me is me liking other people. When we strive to have people like us, we want to feel good about ourselves, which has little to do with the other person. When we strive to like the people around us, it is about them. And for anyone who has experienced being liked, I do not have to tell you the magic of that experience. Fortunately, the common side effect of you liking other people is that many of them will like you!

Let me explain what I mean by liking people. When I know I am going to meet someone new, particularly someone with whom I will be working, I find myself looking forward to the meeting. Usually I have been told a little about the person, and there is a sort of anticipation about meeting him or her. When I do meet this person, that anticipation comes across in the interaction. There is no acting involved; it is just a sincere desire to have this new person come into my life. Based on the reaction of the people I meet, I suspect they feel this anticipation, and I have found almost all respond positively.

Next I find myself interested in learning about the person in front of me. This interest comes from me wanting to know him. Who is he? What is he like? I find myself wanting to know if he likes what he does. How did he become a dentist? If he is from another country, how long has he been here? What was it like to move from one country to another? The curiosity and subsequently the questions that follow are a natural extension of the interest in knowing this new person. In the end, it just comes down to a genuine interest in him.

In the process of getting to know these new friends, as I learn about them, I notice I admire things about virtually each and every one. It might be the dentist who got her dental degree in another country and then had to do it over again here, and the fact that she had that perseverance is inspiring. Or it might be the front desk person who is a single mom and has to take two trains to get to work each day. I find myself asking what kind of person it takes to get up in the morning, take care of a child or children, and then shift gears and walk to a bus stop and use an hour or more of her time getting to work. I just feel what we do as human beings is really very impressive.

When you notice these things, appreciate them, and take a moment to tell people what you admire about them, the most amazing thing happens. People feel seen by you in a way they don't often experience. They generally feel good that someone actually noticed who they are and maybe even cared about them.

Before continuing, I would like to be clear about something. I am not in any way, shape, or form suggesting flattery. Flattery to me is telling someone something that is either an exaggeration, is not true, or is only being said for the purpose of manipulating the other person. No, I am talking about a genuine interest and admiration for the other person. I might say something simple to that front desk person like, "I really don't understand how moms like you juggle everything you juggle." And I'd mean it.

Some people tell me that relating with appreciation in an authentic manner is difficult to do. And I suspect if you see it as a job or something you have to do to achieve a certain result, it probably will be difficult. However, my experience is that learning to genuinely appreciate others is like learning most things. In the beginning, until it is a part of you, it may feel awkward, and then it becomes very natural. Do you remember the first time you rode a bicycle? It was probably awkward. Most likely you were off balance and had to think the whole time. Eventually, however, it became a natural experience that you just *knew* how to do. Learning to express appreciation is very much the same way. In the beginning it may feel awkward, but it soon becomes second nature. Try it one step at a time until it becomes comfortable.

The other concerns I hear from clients are: a) they are uncomfortable saying nice things to people, b) they fear the person will not experience what they are saying as genuine, and c) that people "just don't talk that way." My own experience (and what others who do the same thing tell me) is that just about everyone likes being seen and heard for who they are. Rather than mistrusting, they feel good. If you find yourself uncomfortable noticing and saying positive things to other people, I suspect if you dig deep enough, you will find holding back acknowledgment, praise, and admiration is a learned behavior.

Many of us growing up were taught to hold back and not share our positive feelings about others with them. Worse, some of us grew up in an environment where our caregivers criticized us. Often these caregivers doled out this criticism under the guise of trying to help us correct our flaws by pointing out our weaknesses.[5] This type of help is very detrimental to our wellbeing

---

5 I acknowledge that, from time to time, all of us need feedback that may not be comfortable to hear. In fact, as a coach, I see one of my greatest responsibilities to my clients to be giving difficult feedback and always being honest with them. However, I find I have a lot more I admire about my clients than things I think they should change. Most of my time is spent noticing and telling my clients the things I admire and respect about them. The interesting thing is that when I do tell them about areas that are in their best interests to modify, even when I am strong in the way I tell them, they not only accept the feedback but also seem to appreciate it. I believe this is because they recognize I see them for who they are in both the areas in which they need assistance and the areas in which they excel. If you think about it, when someone criticizes us, we often react negatively to that criticism because we do not feel it fully describes who we are. We feel not fully understood by the person who is criticizing us. I also know that when someone has seen my positive attributes and appreciates them, I tend to have more of a sense that they care about me, and as a result, I am more accepting when they point out the areas in which I need to improve.

and affects our whole lives. Until we become aware and work to change it, this early learning is carried forward into all we do later in life.

In this environment, we learned to focus more on the negatives than positives. From this place, we are trying to avoid receiving that criticism again, so we learn to react. Some might become defiant, others compliant, but in either case, we don't come from our strength. I have a friend whose father would criticize him growing up. He tells a story of when he was fifteen, and he got a B- on a math test. In most cases, he did very well but not in this case. His father came rushing down the stairs to the basement where he was watching TV and yelled, "What is this? Your best is an A. You don't try hard enough." With this type of input, he would work hard to keep his father happy and off his back, and ultimately, he felt he was worthless unless he did well. It took him until his mid-forties to understand and work to change this belief. With his own children, he had to consciously learn to show his appreciation of them. If you have similar stories in your life, then you might have no sense of how to react to appreciation, let alone give it. It takes practice.

You'll find that many of your patients are walking into your treatment rooms with these same stories in their lives. When a medical worker listens to their concerns and appreciates them, it creates an environment they want to come back to. Who wouldn't want that? For example, perhaps you have a phobic patient who has a very strong fear reaction upon entering your treatment room. If you notice he is feeling this way, perhaps you can truly look at this person and appreciate his courage. This experience really scares him, yet he got himself there. The first key is for you to recognize the courage, and the second is to tell him. Perhaps you might say, "You know, I really admire the fact that you're here. I know this isn't easy to do, putting yourself into a situation that feels very difficult. And yet, here you are."

Just be sure you've been able to get to a place within where you genuinely feel that way about the patient. If it is contrived, he'll feel it. With practice, this type of behavior will become second nature to you.

Of course this is not only about your relationships with patients. There is no question that when we are interested in the people we care about, notice their gifts, and tell them what we like about them, they respond positively. For most of us, our default approach is to explain to the people who are close to us what we want from them instead of what we appreciate about them.

How much time do you spend telling your husband, wife, or partner what he or she does wrong or what you think he or she could do better? What kind of reaction do you receive in response? What would happen if you spent most of your time telling that person what you appreciate about him or her?

If there were only one thing I could recommend to dentists about relating to patients, it would be this: like your patients and tell them! Most dentists spend their time trying to get their patients to like them, and that's what comes across. Instead, if you bring all of your attention to being interested in your patients and telling them what you appreciate about them, liking you becomes a nonissue. As we like our patients, an interesting thing happens: they like us back. Patients like and want to be around people who like them. When a patient feels seen, cared about, and respected by you and your staff, it is natural for them to want to come to you.

I recommend starting today to make a consistent effort to notice and appreciate the people around you *and tell them*. I suggest for each criticism you give a staff member, family member, or patient, you give them at least 2.9013 genuine compliments. Yes! 2.9013 to 1, the Losada ratio. A psychologist and consultant by the name of Marcial Losada developed this ratio while studying efficiency in teams.[6] He contends that you need 2.9013 positives to negatives (minimum) to have maximum efficiency. Is there too much of a good thing? Apparently yes. It seems efficiency drops when the ratio exceeds 11.6 to 1. I don't think most of us have to worry about that.

---

6 Achor, *The Seven Principles of Positive Psychology That Fuel Success and Performance at Work*, 60-61.

## Going Deeper

Though it may seem awkward in the beginning, start the process of appreciation one step at a time. These exercises may help you to begin.

1. Carve out some time for yourself when you can become present. Perhaps it's through remembering your just right moment, or perhaps it's through meditation. Close your eyes and think of what you appreciate about yourself. This process may seem unnatural, but it's easier than you think. And it's an important step in learning to appreciate others. What do you like about yourself? What do you do well? Sit quietly with a journal, and write down your thoughts. Be honest and write down only the things you truly feel good about. And don't treat yourself harshly; just being a human being who has made it through to this point, with all the highs and lows, is something pretty wonderful.

2. Pick out a person close to you and practice. Become present first, perhaps through remembering your just right moment or through one of the meditation techniques described above. Think of the person in a positive light, and let your mind focus on what you appreciate about her. What about her do you like? What do you admire? Why do you want to be in her life? Let yourself truly feel this appreciation. Write down these thoughts, perhaps in a list. Set up a time to be with her (or let it happen spontaneously), sit with her, and tell her what you appreciate about her. Pick a new person once a day or once a week until it becomes second nature to you.

3. Pick out a different member of your staff each day, and tell him what you appreciate about him. It can be small or large—the

way he is with patients at the front desk or how he handled a patient during an exam. Be sure you become present first and that you truly believe what you are saying to him.

4. Pick a patient who is on your schedule for that day. In the beginning, it might help to choose a patient you know well. Before meeting with him, sit quietly and list what you appreciate about him. Eventually this might be a mental list, but to start, I recommend that you write it down. Perhaps it's the way he has begun to take care of his teeth over the course of your treatment plan, or perhaps it's his friendly attitude that you noticed during a mix-up in scheduling. It can be small or large, but be clear that you feel genuine about it. When you're with your patient, share your appreciation.

ADRIAN WILKINS

## Hope

*Everything that is done in the world is done by hope.*

—MARTIN LUTHER KING

At the tail end of 2008, when this book had first been conceived, it was a historic time in our country with the election of Barack Obama as president of the United States. Whether you believe that he's been a good or a terrible president, one thing is almost certainly true: at the time of the election, no one since John F. Kennedy had inspired hope in the United States the way this man had. When you consider that Barak Obama is an African American with a middle name of Hussein and was a US senator for less than four years, it is nothing short of a miracle that he was elected to the highest office in the country.

Most people would agree that Obama is smart, hardworking, and articulate. However, there were many smart, hardworking, and articulate candidates in the race for president. And it is true that the backlash against an unpopular president and a collapsing economy worked to his advantage.

However, I am firmly convinced that his message of hope and his ability to communicate that message had more to do with his meteoric rise than any other one factor. Collectively as a country, people made a decision to elect someone during tenuous times who had not yet fully demonstrated his ability to lead. A nation that was already on edge and fearful about its future rejected the status quo in favor of someone who offered them really only one thing. But it is the power of that one thing—hope—that I firmly believe made the difference. I think it has always been true, but now more than ever, we are hungry for hope. Hope just may be the most powerful human force. Without hope, we are capable of very little; with hope, we are capable of almost anything.

What does hope have to do with effective dental communication? As a dentist, you are in a unique position. Many patients enter a dentist's office fearful and perhaps even ashamed of their failing dental health. You have the ability to use that most powerful tool—hope—to alleviate the fear and allow a vision of what's possible to take its place. Your role of sharing this hope in this person's life is special, both because of your realm of expertise and because the person's fear is, in many cases, daunting. One of my clients related a story of a soldier who had been on three combat tours of duty in Iraq. This veteran stated that the single most traumatic event in his life was having his wisdom teeth extracted. Think of that—the level of stress and anxiety that must accompany a single combat tour, let alone three, and his most-traumatic event dealt with dentistry. Your ability to listen to a patient such as this one and engender hope that his experience can be more positive and rewarding will go a long way toward building a powerful and long-lasting relationship.

Once patients feel you like them and care about them, then what they want most from you is hope that their problem can be solved or their desire can be satisfied. If they have dental phobia, they hope their work can be done without fear. If they are in pain, they want to know their pain can be relieved. If they break a tooth, they want to know you can fix it. If they have lots of problems in their mouths and limited resources, they are hoping there is a way to afford the work they need. If they would like a beautiful smile, they want to believe that beautiful smile can be accomplished.

Let's look at an example. My fictitious friend John is frustrated every day as he drives up to the front of his house and sees the lousy state of his yard. He'd love to have one of those *Better Homes and Gardens* lawns, with the bright green grass, the perfectly manicured bushes, and the brightly colored gardens that always make him smile. But his is another story. The grass is burned in most locations and patchy in places where it's green, the bushes are old and dying, and his garden looks a bit like an overgrown compost pile. Season after season, he has tried a few things here and there. He put out the sprinklers but then became too lazy to move them around; he pruned the bushes but perhaps a bit too far; he weeded the garden but only once a season—and each time, he became frustrated and gave up. At least, he thinks, his isn't the worst in the neighborhood. There's Sally's next door. It looks like she did some work in the spring, but it still looks terrible.

Except today, he notices Sally's yard has been transformed: new bushes, bright flowers along the fence line, and grass that's filling in. She even has those pop-up sprinklers that automatically start on a timer. *That must have cost a fortune*, he thinks.

He sees Sally, sucks up his pride, and asks her how she did it. She tells him there's a new lawn care service in town, and to generate interest and get testimonials, they are deeply discounting for a short time. He calls the service, and Bill comes by to hear what John would like. He asks questions about what John would like to see in the lawn, and he listens as John paints the picture of a full lawn, bushes, and a bright garden. John even smiles as he describes it. He discusses his financial needs. Bill understands the yard's current condition and explains what he can do. For the first time since he owned his house, John starts to feel hope that what he wants could be a reality.

In much the same way, in my own work, I am like Bill. I approach my clients with a genuine interest in learning about who they are and what their interests and goals are. I understand where they are now. After getting to know them, I am invariably left with the feeling that there is a solution or at least hope of a solution. This feeling is not the result of a preplanned decision that we will find a way to solve their dilemma. It emerges. I see where they are, I see where they can go, and almost always, a way to get there becomes apparent.

As I move through my own life, I realize I talk to myself in the same way I speak to my clients. Internally I am presented with a challenge and pretty quickly come to the conclusion that something can be done about it. I find myself hopeful that a solution is possible.

If you like your patients and give them hope, I have no doubt they will choose to work with you. Can anyone do this, or is this reserved for the person who naturally likes people and has an innate tendency to be hopeful?

The answer to both questions is yes! Yes, it is more natural for some people than others to be interested in and like the people they meet. Some of us are also born or grow up with a more hopeful approach than others. But it's also true that yes, with a little consciousness and awareness, we can begin to notice how we relate with others and in turn, change how we interact with them.

For example, notice when you meet a patient where your attention is. Do you find yourself interested in who this human being is in front of you? Or instead are you focused on your own thoughts—like the patient respecting you or accepting treatment, or possibly the conversation you need to have with your front desk person later in the day?

As human beings, all of us are at least a little preoccupied with ourselves. We, for all practical purposes, see ourselves as the center of the universe. For most of us, that universe expands outward, first including family and close friends and then the rest of the world. But we see it from our center. It is our nature.

Begin by noticing and recognizing that your patients are also seeing the world that way. Take an interest in their world. Where do they work, do they like it, and is it hard for them to take time out for the dentist? What have been their dental experiences? It really does not matter what you ask—just bring a genuine interest to them. Through this process, you are learning who and where they are. They will naturally reveal their thoughts about dentistry and their past experiences.

Further discussion will lead you to where they want to be. Later we'll discuss in more detail the Comprehensive Exam, and more specifically the Emotional

Exam and how to have these crucial conversations with patients, but at a top level, you are finding out their dentistry wants and needs. Do they want to keep their original teeth? Do they value a less-costly or more-aesthetic solution? Again, the questions don't matter as much as your interest in their universe and their vision of dental health. Like Bill in the example above, he let John share what was important to him, and hope naturally arose.

Most dentists by nature are problem solvers. You meet patients, they present a problem, and you find a solution to their problem. But this approach tends to focus on solving a problem versus understanding the patient. While you must always be honest with the patient, what the patient needs most from you is your confidence that his problem can be solved—not so much for you to solve his problem.

If you pay close attention to what the patient is saying, the challenge or obstacle will become clear. Then it becomes easy to simply help the patient solve his own problem. For example, a patient learns that his treatment will cost around thirty thousand dollars, and he reacts and states, "I can't afford that!" Your natural tendency might be to offer him third-party financing or spread out the payments. But in the long run, it will be more effective to simply give him the opportunity to determine his own solution. Pause… Wait and give the patient time to allow what he is feeling. Oftentimes you will see the patient mentally and sometimes out loud walk through the possibilities when given the opportunity.

Maybe the patient needs a little extra support. You might say, "How could you handle that?" and see how he responds. He will have many more resources to solve his own problem than you can comprehend. He's more familiar with his situation than you. If you give the patient the information and give him a chance to breathe, in most cases, he can solve it himself. By learning where he is and where he wants to be, he has the building blocks for a solution or even a possibility for a solution. And that's more than many would have thought possible. If you support a patient in the areas that he truly wants—be it less fear, a better smile, or both!—then hope is naturally created.

## Going Deeper

How do we grow hope in ourselves so we might support others in their process? Here are a few practices that could support you.

1. Sit and become present with yourself, perhaps through the exercises described in the "Going Deeper" section of "Being Present." Bring to mind an area of your life you feel is impossible to solve. So you can first be comfortable with the process, start with something simple that you don't have a large emotional investment in. Take out a sheet of paper, and write about how it is now—your frustrations, all the ways you've tried to change it. Really write down how it is for you, and get it all on paper. When you think you have it all, take a deep breath and write down anything that's left that you feel needs to be said. Then sit quietly again, letting go of those feelings for the moment.

   Let yourself begin to imagine how you want the situation, process, or way of being to be. Close your eyes, and as best you can, let it come to being in your mind. What does it look like? What does it feel like in this new world of your perfect vision? What could it possibly be like if the situation were perfect for you? Sit with that image for a few minutes, and when it is right for you, turn over the piece of paper and write about what you just imagined—the way it could be. Go into as many details as you can; really get it down on paper. From just this exercise, can you begin to feel hope that there's a possibility of something better? By just allowing a vision of a situation to be different, we naturally feel there are possibilities. Now from this place of how it could be, write down a couple of ways you could get to that vision. Given that you've wrestled with this problem for a while, it may be more difficult to get to, but stay with the vision during this process—that feeling of your vision being reality. Are there more possibilities for solutions when you are thinking of how it could be? Once you feel comfortable with this exercise, you might try one in which you have more emotional investment.

2. Before you see your patients, perhaps at the beginning of the day, review your list of patients and get in touch with a general sense of what you'd hope for the group. Perhaps it is good dental health or a positive experience in this visit. If they are patients you know are especially fearful, perhaps it is that their visits will be calm and peaceful. Though it may sound like a simple thing, if you simply enter the day feeling hopeful, it will change your interaction with them, and there will be more of an opening for them to get in touch with their own sense of possibilities.

## Listen, Listen, Listen

*Better to remain silent and be thought a fool than to speak out and remove all doubt.*

—ABRAHAM LINCOLN

Someone once said to me that he believed in the platinum rule. I corrected him and said, "Don't you mean the golden rule?" The golden rule is, "Treat others as you would like to be treated." He said, "No, the platinum rule. The golden rule isn't bad, but the platinum rule is much more powerful." Of course my curiosity was piqued, and he explained that the platinum rule is, "Treat others as *they* would like to be treated."

We cannot apply the platinum rule until we really understand the other person. To accomplish understanding, we need to listen. Most of us feel cared about when another person listens to us. The way I mean to listen may be a little different from how you have understood it until now. Listening consists of hearing, but it is not limited to hearing. We can hear or we can hear with the purpose of understanding. Hearing is a physical thing, but listening—or what is often referred to as active listening—is a physical, psychological, cognitive, emotional process.

Further, listening as we are using it here includes noticing and integrating body language: things patients do not say, how they dress, how they act, and anything about them that gives you a clue about who they are and what matters to them.

To be an effective listener, you need to have a *genuine interest* in knowing the person to whom you are listening. As stated earlier, human nature is to see ourselves as the center of the universe. Let's face it—I see through my eyes, not yours, I hear through my ears, not yours, and it requires both attention and intention to even attempt to see the world through your eyes.

As someone who has spent his life fascinated by communication, I spend a lot of my time listening. With patient permission, I often listen to recordings of doctors speaking with their patients. Of course, I have the advantage of not being in a real-time conversation, and I'm able to sit back and really listen. But you would be amazed by how often the doctor presenting treatment does not listen to the words and messages the patient is giving and in many cases even interrupts or stops the patient from talking! The following is an example of what can commonly be heard in many dental practices:

Doctor: Hello, Tom. What brought you in today?

Patient: I broke a few fillings and—

Doctor (interrupts): We can definitely take a look at them, and I will tell you how I think I can fix them. Is there anything I should know about you before we take a look?

Patient: No, not really. I just really hope—

Doctor: (interrupts): With all the technology today, it is likely that we can fix them, and if we can't restore your tooth, it is now possible to place implants in place of the extracted tooth. Implants are extremely predictable now. Dentistry has come a long way. In fact, most of the time we are placing implants instead of the treatment that was historically indicated, which was a root canal, post and core, and a crown. It is likely that if your periodontal condition is sound, we will be able to help you to restore your mouth back to health. OK, so it looks like your medical history is normal. Do you have any questions before we go ahead and take a look?

## THE WAY OF THE SUPERIOR DENTIST

Patient: No.

Doctor: OK, let's take a look at what is going on in there.

Though it may be hard to believe, dialogues like the one above are happening every day in dental offices across the country. Now let's try an example of how the dialogue could possibly go:

Doctor: Hello, Tom. What brought you in today?

Patient: I broke a few fillings, and I guess it's time for me to do something about it.

Doctor: Uh huh… Can you tell me a little more about why now?

Patient: Well, I am thinking I shouldn't wait any longer.

Doctor: Uh huh…

Patient: I haven't been in for a while because I haven't taken very good care of my teeth, and now it's been so long, I guess I'm feeling embarrassed.

Doctor: I understand. What kept you away initially?

Patient: Well, I went to someone a few years ago and it really hurt. Plus they wanted to put crowns and implants in, and I didn't want that.

Doctor: Can you say a little more about that?

After listening to the second example, can you guess what might happen if in the first situation the dentist did a typical exam and gave a treatment plan with many crowns and implants? It is really important that we do not talk over patients, and in most situations, saying less is saying more.

Listening, however, does not mean complete silence on the part of the listener. Active listening also includes talking, usually in the form of questions. The intent is to fully understand what the patient means and wants. Open-ended questions often help the patient to provide information that allows the doctor to really understand the patient's needs and wants.

We will explore listening further in part 2, particularly when we discuss the Emotional Exam. In the meantime, let me leave you with this. When I listen to the doctor/patient recordings, I do not have the benefit of facial expressions or body language. As I said, I also don't have any other distractions, but simply by listening, I can hear when patients are anxious. I pick up on their feelings about money, if they feel ashamed, or even if they are telling you yes but saying no, or "I really have no idea what you're talking about." Allowing yourself to truly listen opens up a whole new world of connection, both for you and the person you are interacting with.

For a moment, think about the people in your life you most enjoy talking with. Do they listen to you? Do you leave the conversation feeling that someone heard what you had to say and took in the meaning under the words, responding to the whole of your message? I bet they might even be the people who don't let you get away with anything. You tell them, "Everything is fine," and with a single look, you know they can see through that façade. They absorb your message, not just with their ears. You can provide that same clarity to your patients by listening with all of your senses and responding to all of what is being said, not only the words.

In a way, to truly listen one needs in a nonliteral sense to "get out of the way," to be there as a caring, curious ally to the patient without bringing in any more than necessary our own personal feelings, thoughts, and biases. When we succeed in doing this, patients are able to truly relax, free from our agenda, and are able to explore safely and openly what matters most to them. This listening without judgment or agenda may be one of the greatest gifts one human being can give to another. And for a patient to receive this gift from their health care provider is incredibly rare. Patients virtually always appreciate and value this.

There is another very powerful side effect of this kind of listening. When one person is given this opportunity to think through and express his thoughts, he finds himself becoming clear about what matters to him and what he wants. Have you ever had the experience of going to dinner with a close friend and one of you talks about something that is bothering you and the other one listens? The listener does so without giving advice or interrupting, and at the end the person doing the talking thanks the listener for helping him or her! The person doing the talking starts to have clarity just by being listened to. The person didn't receive advice or a course of action, but all of a sudden things become clear.

The same thing can happen with patients if we really listen to them. We have all been taught our job is to educate, yet most of the time what our patients really need is someone to listen. Because of our desire to provide value to the patients, we spend our time giving information instead of tapping into the wisdom of our patients through listening. For many of the doctors I work with, the switch from educating to listening can often be the crucial piece that allows them to communicate and connect with patients in a way that allows their patients to receive the kind of care they deserve.

## Going Deeper

Active listening, like the other intangibles, is an acquired skill. Practice active listening with people who are close to you and your staff; as your skill grows, you will naturally use it with your patients.

For this listening exercise, first choose a friend or a member of your staff with whom you have a close relationship. This will help you to work through the potentially awkward feelings of this exercise. Here are the rules:

- ❖ Sit across from each other so you can see the other person's body language and expressions.

- ❖ Hold a five-minute conversation in which you only get to ask questions—no statements, just questions.

- ❖ When the person responds, you can ask a follow-up question based only on what the other person states.

For example, the conversation might start something like this:

"How are you doing?"

"Good."

"What has happened that has you saying your day was good?"

"I had a good day at the office and got a few things accomplished that I didn't think I'd get to. And I was able to get something off my chest with my boss."

At this point, you have a choice—do you ask about what the person accomplished or about the conversation with the boss? Depending on what I saw in the other person's body language or voice, I'd follow the thread the other person seemed more interested in. With practice, you will pick up on these cues. Watch facial expressions, whether the voice quickens or the volume increases, and whether the person sits forward or backward. Each of these is a natural indicator of the other person's interest level and comfort with the conversation.

Here are a few ideas to practice during this process:

- Avoid yes/no questions.

- A couple of good leading statements or questions can keep the conversation flowing, such as, "Can you say more about that?"

- Practice pregnant pauses. Let the silence after a question be there so the other person can step into that space and expand on an answer.

- Notice your own reactions during this practice. Do you feel uneasy with asking direct questions? Just noticing will help you to begin to work on your comfort level.

Once you've practiced these conversations a few times, I recommend that you sit with other members of your staff and be both the questioner and the questioned. By getting on both sides of the conversation, you get to experience what it's liked to both listen and be listened to. And if you practice outside the office with those in your life, you may be amazed by how your relationships change for the better!

ADRIAN WILKINS

## About the Intangibles

The intangibles probably account for 90 percent of the success or failure in the doctor-patient communication. Some of us have more natural talent or ability than others; however, regardless of your starting point, everyone can learn to be more present, to focus on appreciating your patients, to provide the hope that your patients are looking to you for, and to listen in a way that allows your patients to give you information you need to help them.

As with many of the things we learn in life, in the beginning, practicing these intangibles may feel awkward and somewhat contrived. But it does not take long before the awkwardness dissolves and you develop a sense of confidence and competence. It really is simply a matter of time, effort, and a bit of courage. When it starts to click, the results are amazing. Patients begin to respond to exactly the same words in a very different way. You may even find yourself asking why they are responding positively now to the same discussions that, in the past, were met with distrust and resistance.

The best part, however, probably has little to do with the result of your patient communication. The best part is how you will feel when you communicate and listen from a place of authenticity. Most dentists describe the experience as energizing and personally fulfilling. This coupled with the fact that these same skills directly translate into an improvement in the quality of your personal relationships makes the effort more than worth it.

In part 2 of the book, we'll look at practical situations and ways each of these concepts can be implemented. For now, we'll turn our attention in chapter 3 to delving more deeply into some of the concepts that are important to effectively communicate this relationship-centered approach. Most patients haven't experienced this approach, so partnering with them becomes very important.

## Summary of Key Points

- *Being Present.* Your ability to be connected to yourself may be the most important thing you can do to connect with your patients.

- *Appreciation.* Keep your focus on what you love about them.

- *Hope.* Be a beacon of possibility for them.

- *Listen, Listen, Listen...* Seek first to understand where they are coming from.

**CHAPTER 3**

# Concepts for Relationship-Centered Dentistry

*Nothing is perfect. Life is messy. Relationships are complex. Outcomes are uncertain. People are irrational.*

—HUGH MACKAY

A friend of mine named Paul needed to have the shower replaced in his house. All the caulking had long peeled away, and the tub stains had begun to look more natural than the original color. They hired a general contractor, Jacob, who joined them at the kitchen table and listened to Paul's interests for this project. He asked Paul, "What's most important to you?" and "How do you want it to look in the end?" Paul was excited about the options in an expensive tub, using his hands to describe how he wanted it to look. Jacob encouraged him to imagine how he'd really like it to be. Paul did so, but then he balanced it against needing to go with an inexpensive shower that included some of his wish list. With these thoughts in mind,

Jacob provided several options, explaining the amount of work required in each, the drawbacks of the cheaper ones, and how each option satisfied the range of interests. Paul and his wife listened intently and picked a cheaper option that had slightly more shelf space than the original tub. They finished their coffee, shook Jacob's hand, and felt good about the interaction.

Jacob purchased and installed the tub but ran into issues with the shower leaking. He informed Paul of what had happened (the type of shower chosen was too cheap and cracked easily), worked with him to have an operational shower while other options were researched, and eventually installed a better-quality tub that was slightly more costly but within Paul's price range. In addition, Jacob ensured that the new tub met more of Paul's needs—it was wider and had even more shelf space—which made the family very happy. Both Paul and Jacob were very satisfied. The key: Jacob partnered with Paul, understanding his needs and desires, and built a relationship up front that helped greatly when challenges presented themselves. He was able to turn a potentially negative situation into a positive for all involved.

I contend that this type of interaction is rare. But when we experience it, it's wonderful, and we remember it years later. It's the type of interaction we want with our patients.

If the intangibles in chapter 2 are the two thousand–foot aerial view, the concepts or operating principles involved in relationship-centered dentistry are more like the view from a second-floor balcony. This next section provides the operating principles for offering comprehensive-care treatment to all of your patients. It makes it possible to do so without scaring those who do not want or cannot afford comprehensive care. It will allow you to treat the ones who do and in the process, give both groups what they need! These principles may seem obvious, but let's talk a little about the benefits of this system.

Of course, one of the primary benefits of this approach is that patients who are interested in comprehensive-care treatment will very often follow through with it—a win-win for the patient and dentist. Many will not do it right away but eventually will end up going forward with most, if not all, of the recommended treatment.

An additional benefit of communicating comprehensive care in a relationship-centered manner is that the patients who are not interested in comprehensive-care treatment are nevertheless well-informed about their situations without feeling pressured by you or your staff. It is my belief that as health care providers, we owe this to our patients. It is not our responsibility to prejudge whether a patient is interested in the best treatment, but only an educated patient is empowered to choose for himself.

## Why Not Decide for the Patient?

*Assumptions are the termites of relationships.*

—HENRY WINKLER

It is natural to make assumptions based on the information we have about what a patient may or may not want to do. At the same time, I regularly hear from doctors about a patient who came in not appearing to have money or a high dental IQ who decided to go forward with extensive treatment. Invariably the doctor will say, "It just goes to show you cannot prejudge." At least until the next time! We all prejudge; it's in our nature. The problem is that it is not fair to the patient and is in fact condescending.

If a patient comes in and if—because of the clothes they are wearing, the job they hold, or some other reason—we do not tell the patient what we see, the implications, and the possible options for treatment, we have not done our job. If because of our preconceived opinion of what he will do or our perception of his financial situation a patient is offered a bridge instead of an implant, or maybe even worse, an extraction instead of the bridge, we are in effect deciding for him.

By deciding for the patients, we are treating them as though they are not capable or do not deserve to decide for themselves. I know this may sound harsh, but to decide for the patient is to treat the patient like a child rather than an adult. With a relationship-centered approach, we are working closely with the patient to assist him in making his own decisions on what treatment is best for him.

My philosophy with comprehensive care is to communicate the benefits and create agreement, never manipulating the patient. With Paul and his shower, he did not feel manipulated; he felt respected, listened to, and a part of the whole process.

One of the important concepts in this approach is to really never present anything. The moment the concept of a presentation is suggested, we are implying a traditional sales process. I will present what I suggest you do, and you will either agree or not agree; if you do not agree, I will convince you of why you should agree. This is not the approach I recommend.

## Co-Diagnosis vs. Presenting or Selling

*The only thing that will redeem mankind is cooperation.*

—BERTRAND RUSSELL

Instead of selling, team up with the patient and create a co-diagnosis and treatment-planning relationship. The advantage to this approach is that there is nothing to sell; the patient ends up owning his situation, and often the patient's knowledge of his own mouth and needs becomes a real asset in creating the treatment plan.

Some dentists can feel a little threatened by this approach. They can feel they are losing control of the process or that maybe the patient will not view them as the experts. My experience has been that patients recognize the confidence it takes for the dentist to be able to put her ego aside and join the patient not as an equal but as part of the team (of patient and doctor) trying to solve the patient's problem.

With the advent of the Internet and all of the information available on the web today, people are much more informed and sophisticated when it comes to their general and oral health than they were twenty years ago. Many patients before walking through the doors of your practice have studied dental implants, cosmetic dentistry, endodontics, and periodontics. I have had more than one dentist tell me of patients coming in to ask them about things that were new to them. The days of a doctor telling the patient what to do and the patient just saying yes are, for the most part, long gone.

Rather than fighting the change, I suggest you embrace it. Give the patient what he wants to the degree that it makes sense. I am not suggesting that you agree to perform treatment you do not feel good about, and neither am I suggesting that you abdicate your role as the expert. I am suggesting that you act more like a teacher, coach, or guide. Side by side with the patient, you provide information and guidance to help him to understand first the situation and then the options. He can then tell you from an informed place which options make sense given his life circumstances.

## Awareness vs. "You Need"

*What is necessary to change a person is
to change his awareness of himself.*

—ABRAHAM MASLOW

This brings us to another important concept. Long before you begin to offer treatment options to a patient, it is crucial that the patient understand he has a problem. This may sound obvious, but daily in thousands of dental offices across the country, the opposite is happening on a consistent basis. I will go so far as to suggest that 90 percent of dentists present treatment directly in contradiction to this important principle.

All you have to do is ask yourself whether you have heard or said any of the following as a way of suggesting treatment to a patient: "Mr. Jones, you need a crown on that tooth," "You need a filling," "You need a root canal," or any other version of "You need." Most dentists I speak with will agree that they either hear this from colleagues regularly or do it themselves.

When treatment is presented this way, an important step is being skipped—that of making a patient fully aware of the problem. A better but not ideal alternative may sound more like this: "You have a cavity, and you need a crown." This is an improvement over the "you need" approach described above in that it makes some effort to explain the problem to the patient. However, it does not fully accomplish the goal of creating awareness with the patient and allowing him to own the problem. The patient's perception of the implications of having a cavity are different depending upon the severity of the cavity and the patient's dental IQ. "You have a cavity and need a filling" can mean different things to different people. Further, because the condition is so closely tied to the solution of needing a filling, it does not allow the patient to easily separate the condition from the solution. This can result in the patient's focus being around the solution and not enough on the condition, the problem, or what he wants.

"You need," or presenting the solution alone or along with the condition, creates another problem. In general we tend to become protective or defensive when we are told we need something. Imagine for a moment you bring your car to an auto mechanic for maintenance. You go to pick up your car and the mechanic says, "You need a new transmission." What is your reaction? Most people feel somewhat distrustful and threatened. After all, your money will be at risk. The natural reaction is to defend, at which point the auto mechanic begins to defend by explaining why you need it. With the defensive nature of both parties already in play, your level of trust and how convincing the mechanic is will determine your course of action. You may go forward, or you may bring the car to someone else.

Consider a different approach, one in which the car owner (or the patient) is involved much earlier in the decision-making process. You arrive at your mechanic to pick up your car from maintenance. The mechanic approaches you and tells you your car is ready and that he would like to show you something. At this point most of us know he is probably going to deliver some bad news, but it does not have the same quality as being told, "You need a transmission."

He lifts the hood and pulls out the transmission fluid dipstick. The fluid is brown. The mechanic shows you the fluid and points out how brown it is. He shows you what red, fresh, clear transmission fluid looks like. Then he smells it and offers for you to do the same, and you notice a burnt smell. He explains that he is concerned because this means the transmission is getting very hot as a result of wear on the metal in the transmission. Then he takes you for a test drive, and as the car shifts, there is a slight lurch as it goes from one gear to the next. He asks if you have noticed that before, and you say yes and tell him you thought it was normal. He continues by explaining that the transmission is jumping from one gear to the next because of wear, which is consistent with the burned transmission fluid. He continues to explain until you understand it as well as a layperson can understand a transmission.

If you are like most people, at some point you ask the mechanic what you can do about it. He explains that if you do nothing, it is a matter of time before the transmission gets worse and breaks down. He then explains that he could drain the fluid and adjust the transmission, but since it has already incurred damage, it will reoccur fairly quickly. Finally, he tells you that he could rebuild or replace the transmission, and he explains the pros and cons of each. He then asks you, "What would you like to do?"

Will you be happy that you need to replace your transmission? Probably not. But will you be as defensive and as likely to go somewhere else? I don't think so. The difference between this and the "You need" approach is that you are involved and educated early in the process; without a solution thrust upon you, you have the emotional space to choose the best solution for you.

How would this look in the case of a crown? "Mr. Jones, I would like to show you what I am seeing when I look in your mouth." At this point, Mr. Jones knows it is probably not good news. He may feel some anxiety, but I contend nowhere near the defensiveness that would occur if you began with, "You need."

Next, utilizing a photograph of his mouth, you show Mr. Jones the large silver filling. You ask him if he notices anything around the edge, and he says yes, he sees a black line all around it. You explain that he is seeing decay, and maybe you even explain what decay is. You explain that the decay is also under the filling. Further, you go on to explain that if the tooth is left untreated, the decay will soon reach the nerve of the tooth, causing pain. Additionally, if still left untreated then, it will eventually result in an abscess and lost tooth. If you allow even just a little space in this conversation, many patients will ask what they can do about it. If not, you can initiate the conversation by saying something like the following.

"You have a few options. You can do nothing and wait until the tooth needs to be removed. Obviously, I do not recommend that. We could also replace the filling, but in your situation, if we do that, there will be so little tooth structure left that the tooth will weaken to the point where it is almost guaranteed to fracture or break off in a short period of time. I really would not feel good about that type of treatment. The best option is for us to take out the old filling, clean out the decay, and cover the whole tooth with a permanent crown that will protect the tooth and is likely to last for years to come. What would *you* like to do?"

When I first suggest this approach, some dentists tell me it seems like a lot of work. This is true; it does take more time to explain things that to you are obvious. However, having commitment versus compliance from the patient is invaluable. And although most dentists initially find dropping the "You need" approach difficult, it does not take long before it becomes second nature.

## The Curse of Knowledge

*Once we know something, we find it hard to imagine what it was like not to know it*

—CHIP AND DAN HEATH

Why do most of us find it more natural to present solutions first? One of the reasons there is a tendency to present solutions instead of educating patients about the condition of their mouths is because it's hard to not know what we know. That's a mind bender, but in essence, we literally cannot imagine what it is like to not understand the ideas and concepts we have mastered, and it is difficult to discuss these ideas with someone else who does not have that same understanding. There is a great discussion of this idea in the book *Made to Stick: Why Some Ideas Survive and Others Die.* In the book, the authors, Chip Heath and Dan Heath, coin a concept called, "The Curse of Knowledge."[7] This concept explains that once we have learned something, especially something we know well, it is difficult for us to recognize and imagine what it is like not to have that information.

In the case of the auto mechanic, when he says you need a transmission, for him it means all of the things explained above. It can actually be difficult for that mechanic to realize you do not have that knowledge.

When you talk to a patient about needing a crown, it is first difficult to remember the patient may or may not know what is meant by a crown in this context. If one dentist is speaking to another dentist and says he needs a crown, it is obvious to both that the patient most likely has decay and that the tooth is not sound. Further, it means if the decay is left untreated, eventually it will reach the nerve, and then if still left untreated, it will cause pain and the eventual loss of the tooth.

For the dentist the words, "You need a crown" include in their meaning all of the above. In saying this statement to the patient, the dentist is really saying, "There is decay in your tooth. That means that the hard surface of the tooth called the enamel is compromised. Decay occurs when bacteria causes the breakdown of the chemical composition of the tooth surface. When this happens, if it is left untreated, it will eventually spread through the soft inner part of the tooth and finally reach the nerve and kill the nerve. If we wait for that to happen, there will be pain, additional cost for treatment, and often even a loss of the tooth."

Depending upon the dental IQ of patients, they may or may not understand all of this when you tell them they need a crown. But for the dentist, it is difficult to imagine people do not know something that appears to you as simple and obvious as this.

---

7   Heath, *Made to Stick: Why Some Ideas Survive and Others Die*, 46, 57.

This communication problem becomes much greater when we start to talk about needing an implant or a root canal. The doctor shortens the explanation of the condition, consequences, and treatment into just a shorthand discussion of the needed treatment.

This problem also happens because the dentist often believes the patient is not interested in knowing the details of the condition and its implications. From her perspective, the patient just knows there is a problem and should accept the recommended treatment. Sometimes this is true, but as we will examine later, even when we know for certain the patient is not interested, we are still better off explaining the situation. By informing the patient, you are gaining commitment rather than compliance.

There are even some dentists who feel insulted that the patient expects to be told conditions and consequences. The feeling is, "Why doesn't the patient just trust me?" This is about the dentists' ego and has no place in the type of co-diagnosis we are advocating here.

## Fear of Scaring the Patient

When discussing the concept of comprehensive examinations and a full-mouth education, many dentists share a major concern. They are concerned the patient will be overwhelmed, not trust the dentist, and in some cases leave the practice because they are afraid they are being "sold."

These same dentists will often tell me that when they meet a patient who has a lot of needs, they will avoid telling the patient about all of the problems. This approach typically begins with telling the patient about some minor treatment so the patient will get comfortable with the dentist and ends with either avoiding the other needs or telling the patient, "Let's start here, and we will talk about the rest later."

I understand the intention behind this approach, but it is a serious mistake. Instead of having the intended consequence, it often accomplishes just the opposite and results in the patient not trusting the dentist.

## Trust

*To be trusted is a greater compliment than being loved.*

—GEORGE MACDONALD

With this approach, the dentist is intentionally withholding important information about the patient that he deserves and needs to establish trust. Think about that. We avoid telling the patient the whole truth to build and create trust. In the best light, the purpose is to not overwhelm and to show the patient you will not push him. In the worst light, it is avoidance of the situation because the dentist is out of integrity with herself and believes the goal is to sneak up on the patient and get him to do it later.

What most of us tend to forget or ignore is that in general, people pay more attention to the intention of our energy than to what we say. Communication specialists state that anywhere from 60 to 90 percent of the message in an interaction is nonverbal. What we say is nowhere near as important as what we believe when we are saying it. This situation is why being present is so important.

Human beings have an amazing ability to pick up on tone, body language, cadence, etc., in judging the intention of a person speaking to us. Most of us believe we can tell when someone is being straight with us. It has been my experience that most of us also think we are better at fooling the other person than we really are. This is because the other person doesn't tell us he or she does not believe us. It is impolite and too confrontational. So when a dentist is holding back information, going slowly and telling the patient about something small, and waiting on telling the really bad news until after she's built a relationship, the patient feels something is off. He may not know for sure what it is and may not even be fully conscious of his suspicion, but nonetheless he is suspicious at some level.

The next problem develops when the patient comes back in six months or a year for his next exam or hygiene check. How does the dentist now tell the patient about the conditions she did not tell him about the first time? Some dentists keep finding reasons to put off telling patients or they tell them about one tooth at a time, and the patients really begin to lose trust. Each time they come, it is something else. In the end, the original objective of building trust on top of a deception can never work.

Most people would agree that the way to build trust (and the way they would like to be treated) is just the opposite of what is described above. Most would say that the way to build trust is to tell the truth even if it risks having the other person be upset with us. By telling others the way it really is, the other person develops confidence that what we are saying is true.

The same is true when we are presenting conditions and treatment needs to a patient. The patient may not like getting the bad news, but the trust that is created by telling it like it is becomes the foundation for future interactions.

The holding back information approach is ineffective, but there is an element of wisdom in the desire to go slowly with a patient. The wisdom comes in recognizing that patients get overwhelmed and are often afraid of the news they receive from their dentist. Many have also had experiences of a dentist pressuring them to accept "optimal dental care" as defined by the dentist. It is no surprise that they are leery of someone telling them about extensive needs and treatment. The fear is that they will be pushed to do everything the dentist says they should do.

However, the solution is not to hold back information from the patient until the "right time." Rather, the solution is to explain to the patient that in his situation, there are a number of options, and he will have some decisions to make. Your goal is to explain it to him so he understands the situation and the implications of the conditions present and also assure him that he will be in complete control of what to do about it. Period. No judgment, no pressure, nothing.

People in general are not scared away by getting information, even if that information suggests to them they need extensive work. But even the smallest amount of treatment, even a small filling, can cause patients to be upset or frightened if they question the necessity of the work through lack of trust.

## The Ostrich

*Denial ain't just a river in Egypt.*

—MARK TWAIN

Are there patients who do not want the information? Yes, of course. There will always be the patient who does not want radiographs, does not want you to check for oral cancer, and certainly does not want to hear about potential dental needs. These people avoid problems the way an ostrich buries its head in the sand. This behavior isn't limited to dentistry and is how they deal with other problems in life. Any effort to educate or explain will most likely be met with resistance.

With these types of patients, there is probably very little you can do. If they stay in your practice, it is even more important than normal to educate them and document the fact that you have done that. In most practices, however, this kind of patient will leave you and try to find a dentist who will collude with them in ignoring the problems.

I do not generally subscribe to the attitude of dismissing patients who do not fit within a strict parameter. I believe as dental health professionals, our goal should be to educate as many people as possible about comprehensive care and meet them where they are. The patient who truly has no desire to even know what is going on is probably one of the few types for whom the approach in this book will not serve. The good news is that it's not a common problem.

However, if you do run into one of these types of patients, what you can do is let these patients tell their story, and perhaps they will not be ostriches after all. At times, before a patient can connect with you, he needs to get his past experiences with dental care out of his system. Much like you as a practitioner, a patient needs to find ways to be present. If he is consciously or unconsciously holding back, there is no way to build trust, and what may seem like a patient who doesn't want to know is merely a patient who does not want to confront his own fear. In this case, invite the patient to tell his story. Think of the times in your life when you've held back from telling a spouse or a friend something you didn't think they wanted to hear or wouldn't understand. If you're like many people, you'll hold back or even avoid this person and maybe even blame him or her for you not being able to speak what is true for you. Then one day you get the courage to state what you're truly feeling, and it's like an old room that has been closed up for winter that finally has the windows opened and the warm breeze of spring let in. Trust can grow. The same is true with many of your patients. Many of us grew up with dentists who simply told us what to do, didn't pay attention to our fears or pain, and barreled on through.

For example, a friend's father once told him this story of going to the dentist: "I went to a dentist because I had three teeth that were very painful and needed to be pulled out. I hate going to the dentist, but this really needed to be done. I told him that I wanted to be knocked out, and he said, 'OK, lie back,' and he gave me Novocain. I said, 'Really, Doc, I want to be knocked out.' He said, 'Lie back.' I did, and he reached into my mouth and pulled the three teeth. I couldn't believe it." Whether the dentist was right or wrong medically, how could this person ever trust this dentist again? You have people every day with these experiences walking into your office. What may seem like an ostrich may really be a person who felt an incredible breach of trust.

It is absolutely true that some people just don't want to know, despite your best efforts. These patients should be respected for their position and perhaps told you can't treat them. But some just need to get their stories out so they can build a relationship with you. Let them.

## Educating Patients

*When a person is down in the world, an ounce of help is better than a pound of preaching.*

—EDWARD G. BULWER-LYTTON

Does educating patients really work? Yes, once they want to know the information. The mistake most dentists make when they try to educate patients is that they try to give patients information they are not yet interested in receiving.

The key to educating patients is to give them information that is relevant to them. Imagine for a moment that you are on an airplane ready to take off. The pilot comes on the intercom and tells you that the flight attendant is going to give you the safety instructions for the flight. You find yourself watching and listening a little, but for the most part you are engaged in your magazine or talking to the person next to you. The flight attendant is not very successful in educating you or most of the people on the plane because the information is not very relevant to you in that moment.

Now imagine you are at thirty thousand feet and the pilot comes on the intercom and explains they are having engine trouble and are turning around for an emergency landing. Just to be safe, he is going to ask the flight attendant to go over the safety instructions again. Now what are the chances you and the others on the plane will really listen? The information that the flight attendant is going to deliver now is very relevant. Now the more information and the more detailed the information the better.

The point is to educate patients on what they want and what is relevant to them. With the rare exception of the true ostrich, educating patients will not drive them away. But how you do it can. Here are some keys to making patients aware of their situation.

## Expectations

*If you paint in your mind a picture of bright and happy expectations, you put yourself into a condition conducive to your goal.*

—NORMAN VINCENT PEALE

First, patients need to know what to expect. It is easy to lose sight of what the dental experience is like for a new patient in a typical examination. With the exception of some very unusual people, most of us feel threatened when we do not know what is going to happen.

If the dentist is examining a new patient, it is typical that the patient has just filled out paperwork, had radiographs and hopefully photographs taken, and received a periodontal charting, a tooth charting, and an occlusion evaluation, among others. Most of it has taken place with people he has just met while he is in a vulnerable, reclined position. Just knowing what is going to happen, how long it will take, and exactly what to expect can go a long way toward lowering the patient's apprehension.

Patients also worry about what they are going to be told and what they will need. I recommend telling the patients up front that you will give them an overall idea of what is going on, but you will have them come back after you have studied their situation, and together you will decide what to do. I would further reassure them that regardless of what you find, there will be no pressure for them to accept treatment. In addition, they will have plenty of time to consider what, if anything, they would like to do about what you find and when they would like to do it. If you tell patients in advance what will happen in the exam, reassure them that there will be plenty of time to decide what to do, and let them know the next steps, rarely, if ever, will you scare them away. The bottom line is to let the patients stay in control.

## Control

*Yeah, {going to the dentist is} a little difficult for me, because of what had happened to me in the past. I just get that feeling...when you have no control because you're in the chair, your mouth is frozen, and you're pretty much at the mercy of that person.*

—A MALE SURVIVOR OF CHILD SEXUAL ABUSE [8]

---

8 Stalker, Carruthers, Teram, & Schachter, "Providing Dental Care to Survivors of Childhood Sexual Abuse: Treatment Considerations for the Practitioner," 1277.

*{The dentist} tells me what he's going to do next. So, long before I can anticipate, he's already told me...* [9]

It's important to be mindful that there is an inherent power disparity between the doctor and the patient, and this disparity can easily put the patient on the defensive. This inequality comes from both the patient's lack of dental knowledge (i.e., he can't have a peer-to-peer discussion with you on the benefits of an implant over a bridge for missing teeth) and his vulnerability associated with having his mouth touched and manipulated.

In a 2005 *Journal of American Dental Association* article, from which the above quote was taken, the authors state that given the prevalence of sexual abuse in the general population, a dentist likely sees patients with such an experience several times a week. From their research, "reliable evidence indicates that up to 13 percent of females and between 5 and 10 percent of males have been exposed during childhood to acts of sexual abuse that involved penetration." [10] That means roughly one in eight female patients and between one in ten to twenty male patients has experienced a severe form of abuse. For these patients, even the most basic dental practices can be triggers, including reclining in the dental chair and bodily touch.

Though they may be more sensitive to these situations, it's not just sexual abuse survivors who feel this discomfort. Most of us have some level of anxiety with uncertain circumstances that may involve pain and require us to trust another in a vulnerable position. So what is a dentist to do?

---

9  Ibid, 1280.
10  Ibid., 1277.

As you learned in dental school, within certain parameters, let the patient know he will have control over his treatment. No one will make him do anything. Explain that your job is to be the technical expert and you will pass that expertise on to him as it relates to his oral health. Then together you will decide what is right for him. Does this mean you give up your role as the expert? No. Does it mean you perform dentistry you do not believe in? Again, no. But you can work together with the patient.

While performing clinical work, be present with what is happening with your patient. Is he tense? Did his demeanor change during different parts of the procedure? If so, then some of the techniques described by survivors may help. Asking permission to continue with a procedure can help lower fear. And a practice of "Inform before You Perform" can build trust. As one patient stated, "I find her good because she does explain everything that she is going to do and why she's doing it at the time and sort of checks, 'Is that OK?'"[11] In some cases, if the patient seems especially nervous, you might establish a hand signal to allow him more control over when you should stop.

At the more strategic level, when performing comprehensive exams and reviews of findings and determining specific treatments to perform, ultimately all patients need to be responsible for their own health, whether that is a choice to smoke or not smoke, drink or not drink, exercise or not exercise, or keep a tooth or have it extracted. But by being aware of the wide range of fears that people bring into your offices and consciously partnering with them, you can better serve them. Allow the patient to be a part of the process.

---

11  Ibid.

## Should vs. Want

*All that spirits desire, spirits attain.*

—KHALIL GIBRAN

I run an exercise in my workshops where I ask all the participants to think of something in their lives they should do. They list them out, and invariably, someone will bring up losing weight. I ask the person why he should lose weight, and he'll say, "It's better on the knees and my heart," or some such. I then ask him, "If I bring in a famous doctor who tells you all the other reasons why you should lose weight, and I give you a bunch of articles, would that convince you to make the decision?" The person then laughs and says no.

Ultimately, the person will lose weight because he wants to lose the weight, not because he's been educated to do so. The person likely already knows the many reasons he should. It really comes down to his wants. Yet we educate our patients all the time on their "shoulds." It won't help them choose the best care. Instead, spend the time understanding what your patient wants. You'll be much more effective in educating him on how he can fulfill those wants rather than trying to educate him around things he already knows he should do.

## Cost and Trust

*The cost of a thing is the amount of what I will call life which is required to be exchanged for it, immediately or in the long run.*

—HENRY DAVID THOREAU

We have already discussed patient awareness as a key component to building a successful relationship. However, I cannot stress enough the importance of explaining in detail what is happening and what it means to the patient. It is especially true as it relates to communicating comprehensive treatment plans and building trust. The key question is, "Who should the patient trust?"

If a patient needs a small filling and his insurance will pay for 80 percent of the cost, it is not difficult for him to say yes. He probably understands what decay is (although I suspect many do not even know in advance which tooth is being filled), and even if he is not sure he needs it, so what? The insurance company is paying for most of it, he does not want to be a noncompliant patient, and it is easier just to say yes.

But as treatment becomes more complicated and expensive and has greater health implications, patient education becomes more important. Telling a patient he needs a full-mouth reconstruction is not the same as telling a patient he needs a one-surface composite.

When a procedure is low in cost and implications, it can easily be recommended based on minimal explanation and minimal trust. As a procedure becomes more complicated and expensive, the trust is stretched, and patient education and awareness become critical.

But we tend to focus on the idea of patients trusting us instead of trusting themselves. The dependence on patients trusting in the doctor to create agreement for treatment has an inherent number of issues. One of the biggest problems is that trust is dependent on the person trusting, not the person trying to be trusted. How does one person make another trust her? She can't. The dentist can only create the conditions that might allow a patient to choose to trust her. If the patient has problems with trust or has had other bad experiences, trusting this dentist will be a problem. It is true that we can create an environment that fosters trust, and the approach being put forth here often does that. However, it is still up to the patients to decide to trust, and no matter what you do, they may never feel comfortable doing that.

The other problem is that sometimes we are successful in gaining full patient trust, and that can lead to bigger issues. I am talking about the patient who puts all his faith in the dentist. The words that concern me the most in a Review of Findings appointment are, "Whatever you say, Dr. Brown. I trust you."

It is great that the patient trusts Dr. Brown, but it is a real problem that the patient is basing his full treatment decision on his trust in her. If you are Dr. Brown, initially it might feel good to be trusted by the patient, but often immediately following that good feeling is a sense of burden and pressure for the treatment to go well.

Who do you think responds better to a failed procedure—the patient who understood why he was having the procedure and did it because he wanted to do it or the patient who really did not understand but trusted his doctor?

It is always better to have the patient choose treatment because he understands he has a problem. He owns the problem, understands the implications of having it, has received options, and is allowed to choose the option that suits him best without pressure. With this information and the space to make a decision, the patient trusts himself, and that's where the trust belongs.

The level of trust a patient will exhibit is often evident in his personality. We will explore personality types in this book, but for now it is important to know that people do respond differently to the concept of co-diagnosis and oral health awareness. To some extent, these differences impact the level of detail and the interest of the patients to engage in learning about their situation. Some patients want to know every detail and what it means to them. With this type of patient, education is easy, and you will most likely be able to help him understand what is happening in his mouth.

Other patients by nature will be more focused on their relationship with you and others in the office. They may not care as much about understanding how an implant integrates with the bone. This is the kind of patient who is likely to say, "I trust you, Doc." However, even with this patient, it is important to explain the situation to the extent he is willing or able to hear it. The key is to make the information relevant because the patient is much more likely to want to be informed if it's relevant to his question. The more a patient understands what is going on, the more likely you are to have a positive relationship with him, regardless of whether he does or does not choose comprehensive-care treatment.

## Speak in Layman's Terms

*You must learn to talk clearly. The jargon of scientific terminology which rolls off your tongues is mental garbage.*

—MARTIN H. FISCHER

"I found the problem with your computer system, Dr. Smith. There are several issues we'll need to take care of. Since AD is running on the file server, I took a look there first. Your LDAP bind time is pretty high, and the pages/sec was well over twenty. Your available bytes are very low, too. I also noted that your cache bytes are well over four MB, and your current disk queue length is over three. And that's just on the DC! Your VM is sized correctly, and I did run the PM remotely, so that didn't affect the results. All of this is keeping the PCs from authenticating to the DCs and your apps from accessing the DBs. What I'm getting at, Dr. Smith, is that you'll need to buy a new server, make DC1 into DC2, replicate AD, and you'll be all set. It'll cost around five thousand dollars to get it done."

Sounds crazy, right? And though the example is pretty extreme, I have seen similar dentistry-related language from my clients. One of the most common mistakes I have seen dentists make in presenting treatment is the use of technical jargon. More often than you might believe, I hear things like, "Mr. Jones, on numbers thirty and thirty-one there is severe periodontitis with furcation involvement." Or "Mr. Jones, the first thing we are going to do is open your bite and facilitate the correct occlusion. In order to do this we will perform a sinus lift, a bone graft, and an implant. When the bone integrates, we will restore the teeth."

I am not exaggerating. Usually at this point, if I am present for the appointment, I watch the patient's eyes glaze over. He has that look most of us have on Thanksgiving Day after too much turkey and too much alcohol, when the football game and the fire are about to put us to sleep. If I am listening to a recording of the appointment, there is often a quiet pause and possibly a couple of "uh-huhs" from the patient. Once in a while, I hear a bold-faced lie that comes in the form of, "I understand, Doctor."

I may not be the first person to suggest that you avoid technical jargon. When we hear stories like the one above, we generally laugh and recognize the absurdity of it. But even when people tell us, we have a tendency to speak in terms that make sense to us and mean little or nothing to the patient. I once had a doctor client who could not help using technical jargon in his Review of Findings appointments. I took one of his recordings and dubbed in the words "blah, blah, blah" in place of each technical term. When he first listened to it, he was stunned by how little the patient could possibly understand based on what he was doing. As he listened a little longer, he burst into laughter when he realized how absurd it was.

If it is not helpful, then why do we do it? It's not just limited to medicine. In any field that has technical language specific to that field, you will find members of that field speaking in technical terms. There are a few reasons.

The first is what I referred to earlier—the curse of knowledge. It is not easy to remember that what we know others do not know. It's as simple as that. We have forgotten that someone once defined for us the terms we are using. Now it is a shortcut, and each time we need to communicate that concept, using these terms is more efficient than speaking all of the words that define that term.

It makes sense and is perfectly reasonable, but it is a problem in communication for a couple of reasons. The first reason is the obvious one in that the patient does not understand what you are talking about. The second is related but slightly different. People often make decisions for emotional reasons. It's the reason you'll see charity organizations putting up pictures of individual children to sponsor; they know people are more likely to decide to donate if there is an emotional connection. Your patients are trying to decide their course of action, and speaking in technical terms puts the patient's mind in an analytical mode instead of an emotional mode. This is further exacerbated by the patient trying to figure out what is being said and using the problem-solving part of his brain. If you speak in terms patients understand, they are more likely to stay present with you and the decisions they need to make.

There is another reason professionals use technical terms. Ego. The conscious or unconscious thinking is to impress the patient with how much you know so he will think you are the right person to perform the work. Some dentists even do it to intimidate the patient and attempt to make themselves feel bigger, and in turn the patient smaller, to create a power disparity. This comes from a lack of self-esteem and a need to feel important. Generally this lack of self-esteem is obvious to everyone but the person doing it. Whether in dentistry or another field, you probably can remember times when you listened to someone spout off and wondered the whole time if he knew what he sounded like.

Sometimes it seems to work, at least to some degree. The patient may be impressed, yet he often feels inferior to the doctor. This can result in the doctor looking like she knows what she is talking about, but it almost always comes at the cost of the patient's self-esteem.

In all situations, it is better to speak to the patient in his language, not yours. If you met people from China and you spoke both Chinese and English and they only spoke Chinese, you would speak Chinese to them. You would not speak English in the hope of impressing them or talking down to them.

Since you speak Layman and also dental technical language and most of your patients primarily speak Layman, speak Layman. Listen in your mind over and over as you speak, and take out every single dental term. The hardest ones to change are the simplest ones; you use them over and over, and you really have forgotten that your patients don't know them.

Some examples:

| Dentist's Terms | Layman's Terms |
| --- | --- |
| *Lingual/palatal* | *Tongue side/cheek side* |
| *Fracture* | *Crack* |
| *Occlusion* | *The bite/how teeth come together* |
| *Tooth numbers* | *Left back molar* |
| *Sub gingival* | *Below the gum line* |
| *Posterior/anterior* | *Back teeth/front teeth* |
| *Mandible/maxilla* | *Lower/upper teeth* |

And the computer problem above? The technician is detecting that the system has become overloaded and is running slowly. He recommends that you buy a new server and keep the old one to help balance the load. It'll cost a bit to do, but in the long run, it will serve your growing business well.

## Analogies, Metaphors, and Similes

*When an analogy is really singing, it's what you want it to be.*

—ETHAN HAWKE

A colleague of mine stated to a client, "Sam, you're ready to go all out in your life, but you don't believe it. It's a little like you're out on a racetrack on a tricycle. Your racecar is right there, but you're choosing the tricycle."

That simple image stopped the client in her tracks and gave her a different view of how she was approaching her life. It was powerful enough for her that months later, she still used it, saying, "Oh, I'm choosing the tricycle again." That's the power of analogies and metaphors: they can quickly bring into focus a somewhat difficult idea.

The language of images, stories, and comparison is not new to dental communication. Since the beginning of dentistry, doctors have been explaining conditions and proposed treatment with analogies and metaphors.

As we discussed above, technical jargon is confusing and dry. It immediately puts people into an analytical state of mind, which, unless the patient is looking for technical speak, is generally ineffective. Comparisons that make sense to patients in their world tend to be more effective in communicating a concept. Speaking to a patient in his lingo is speaking to him in his "language of impact."

The language of impact can be general or specific. For example: "With this old silver filling, the more you chew, it is as though the filling is being pounded into the tooth the way you would pound a wedge into a piece of wood. Eventually the wood—or the tooth in this case—will split." Almost anyone can understand this analogy, and it is likely to have impact. The more specific you can make it to the person, the better; this example would have an even a greater effect with a carpenter or logger.

I recommend that you look for the language of impact for each of your patients. In most situations you can you use the same expressions, but the more you can meet people on their own turf, the better. Practice using images, stories, and comparisons in all of your dental communication. A laser cavity detector focuses your attention to problem areas of the mouth; in a similar way, use of analogies and metaphors will go a long way toward focusing your patient's attention to specific ideas you're hoping to communicate.

## Going Deeper

1. Developing your own analogies, metaphors, and similes can help you to communicate with your patients. For this exercise, pick three of the conditions below, and develop metaphors you can use to explain this problem to a patient.

    a. Lack of bone due to periodontal disease

    b. How a crown protects a tooth

    c. Need for crown lengthening

    d. Deep scaling

    e. Root canal

2. As a further exploration, write down your own problems and conditions and develop analogies, metaphors, and similes that will help you to describe them.

3. Practice what you've created with your staff to see if it helps to get the ideas across. If so, begin to sprinkle them into your conversations with your patients.

ADRIAN WILKINS

# Identify the Patient's Objectives

*Begin with the end in mind.*

—STEPHEN COVEY

One of the most crucial steps regularly missed in reviewing treatment, or in any patient interaction, is finding out what matters to the patient. I can't emphasize this enough. From the first phone call, other than being fully present, there is nothing more important to effectively communicating with a patient than understanding his goals and objectives. The mistake most of us make is assuming we know what is important to the other person. Unfortunately, our tendency is to determine that based on what is important to us. Remember the Platinum Rule—treat others as they would like to be treated.

You believe all people should want to keep all of their teeth for a lifetime, but that does not mean your patient feels the same way. Perhaps he believes he would look better in dentures. It may be true that if you explain to a patient the health and overall impact of ending up in dentures, he most likely will decide he wants to keep his teeth for a lifetime. But you can't have a trusting dialog with the patient until you know what he's thinking. If you don't know, it's a little like playing a blindfolded game of pin the treatment on the patient. Nobody is served in that situation. You need to begin on the same wavelength, understanding and accepting the patient's point of view.

I held a coaching session with a dentist who had just completed a meeting with a patient. The dentist looked a little uncomfortable and sheepishly explained to me that he had not done a very good job in the appointment. He went on to explain that he had discussed all the details of his findings with the patient, but he had not placed a lot of emphasis on the whys of considering treatment. Apparently this patient, in his mid-thirties, had just lost his job, and his wife of the same age was dying of cancer. He explained to the dentist that he realized he had some problems, but right now all he could deal with was keeping a roof over his sick wife's head.

I reassured the dentist that in my mind, he had done the exact right thing. He listened to what was important to the patient and acted accordingly. How do you talk about the value of a beautiful smile or the potential of losing teeth when this is clearly not the patient's biggest priority?

This is a perfect example of putting one of the intangibles into action. I do not think anything helps human beings feel more important or cared about than a genuine interest on the part of another to understand them. Always remember, there is a person behind the teeth.

Ask your patients what is important to them. Are they interested in a Brad Pitt/Angelina Jolie smile? How do they feel about dentures? Is the priority to stay out of pain? Is it to keep their teeth for a lifetime? What is their time/money budget? Is this a good point in their lives to take the next step in terms of their oral health?

How can we possibly speak to a patient about treatment without understanding his objectives? When I say this, some dentists become concerned that patients cannot know what they want until they have been educated. There is certainly wisdom behind this concern. But I contend that you can't know what to educate them on until you know what they want. How could you? If you walked into a shoe store and the salesperson started telling you about the latest sneakers when you really wanted dress shoes, she's wasted your time. You'll find that determining what is and isn't relevant will be a back-and-forth dance with the patient. As you learn what patients want and begin to educate them based on both that knowledge and what you're seeing in the exams, you can then effectively communicate with them.

These objectives will grow and change over time and with the information you provide. A patient may tell you cost is the number-one objective until he realizes that the solution is extracting a tooth instead of saving it. Goals and objectives are not static.

When the patient says, "Now that I understand the implications of losing a tooth, I don't want to lose it," it is simply a matter of saying to the patient, "I understand, and we can look at doing that. I mentioned the extraction based on your concern about cost. I now hear that you still care about the cost but not losing the tooth is a priority as well. This is what I suggest…" Because of new information, the patient changed his objective, and the dentist modified her suggestion.

As I describe this approach, it probably sounds obvious. Listen to what the patient wants, and give it to him. It's so obvious that one has to wonder, why would anyone do anything else? What stops us? I say most of us have an agenda in our interactions with another person. What I mean by "agenda" is that we want a specific outcome or result to come from our interaction. In and of itself, there is nothing wrong with having an agenda. Part of the reason you are a dentist is that you want to make money. Making money is an agenda. When you talk to a patient about his condition and possible treatment, at some level, you probably have an agenda about making money.

The problem arises when we are not conscious of our agendas or we try to hide or force our agenda on the other person. For example, what do we do when our personal values or the type of dentistry we want to perform is in conflict with the goals and objectives of the patient? This happens all the time. It can be something as simple as a patient who refuses radiographs. Or it can be deeper, that you have a personal/professional value about not extracting teeth or not making dentures, yet the patient wants dentures. Clearly, you have an agenda, the patient has an agenda, and they are in conflict.

First seek to understand the patient's agenda. Why doesn't he want radiographs? Is it cost? Is it radiation? Is it a fear of finding out something is wrong? Once you understand why, address the issue honestly with him. If after you have done that, you feel you cannot treat him, tell him that without judgment, and set him free. What is important here is to explore and understand first, and then if what the patient wants violates your ethical standards, explain that without anger or judgment. When it is done this way, most patients understand and appreciate the honesty.

In a case where the type of service you want to provide differs from what the patient wants, again, it is a matter of listening, explaining, and then together recognizing the relationship is not a good fit. Just because you believe implants are the standard of care does not make the patient wrong for choosing a denture. However, deciding to place implants and not dentures is always your choice. The problem stems from imposing our values and beliefs upon the patient. And when we succumb to this unspoken agenda, the results are usually disastrous. The dentist is frustrated, the patient does not feel seen or heard, and the trust between the doctor and patient is damaged.

Remember, listening is one of the most valuable intangibles of success. I suggest that in an effective Emotional Exam, Clinical Exam, or Review of Findings appointment the doctor should speak less than 40 percent of the time and more like 20 to 25 percent! The majority of the time should be spent with the patient doing the talking.

Conveying technical information to the patient is the least-important part of your appointments. Hearing what the patient is trying to say and what matters to him, and ensuring he understands, is where you create all of the value.

## Patient Anxiety

*{When I think about going to the dentist,} to be honest with you, I'm a little nervous, even if it's just to get a teeth cleaning. I've been nervous because of all the work I had done when I was younger. I'm*

*afraid they'll find something I need work on, and in the past, they all involve some form of pain.*

—FORTY-FIVE-YEAR-OLD WOMAN

*I am twenty-four years old and have to have my front teeth pulled today. The dentist prescribed me {valium} but I am still scared so bad that my stomach is starting to hurt. I have tried the gas but I freaked out so I doubt that's an option. I have really bad anxiety and don't know if I can go through with it...*

—TWENTY-FOUR-YEAR-OLD MAN [12]

*I don't like going to the dentist. I don't like the part when they put the gross stuff all over your teeth. It tastes gross. And when they scrape my teeth, sometimes they miss and get my gums. And that hurts.*

—NINE-YEAR-OLD GIRL

In 2003, Dr. Brian Chanpong and members of the Toronto Faculty of Dentistry set out to determine the demand for sedation for patients in Canada.[13] During this process, they reviewed available literature worldwide and found that between 4 and 20 percent of the population reported high

---

[12] Anonymous, *I go to the dentist today and am so scared?*
[13] Chanpong, Haas, & Locker, "Need and Demand for Sedation or General Anesthesia in Dentistry: A National Survey of the Canadian Population," 3-4.

levels of dental anxiety. In the United States, surveys showed between 10 and 19 percent had a similar high-anxiety level. In 2007, Dr. Chanpong, with additional associates, continued this research and found that more than 50 percent of patients reported at least some level of anxiety.[14] It is true that studies of fearful patients' perception of the pain they would experience was generally greater than what they actually experienced, but in a way, that doesn't really matter. What matters is the patient's perception when he walks into your exam room.

During all appointments, it is very important to explore this anxiety. I know that to most dentists, this statement may seem obvious. However, most clinicians, even though they know many people are anxious, do not adequately investigate this issue, and worse, they often discount it when the patient brings it into the discussion. I believe this is because dentists have become so desensitized to the number of phobic patients that it becomes difficult to see something that is constantly around them. Further, it can feel daunting to try to deal with all of these fearful patients, so it is easier to want to believe it is less of an issue than it really is. But patient anxiety or fear is present for many more of your patients than the ones who acknowledge it openly.

Most likely for reasons related to embarrassment or pride, many patients will not volunteer their fears. In fact, many of them will consciously hide the issue, making it a challenge for the dentist to recognize the problem. To make matters worse, quite often these patients will avoid treatment. Many have not taken care of their mouths, have not visited the dentist recently, and are in need of extensive treatment. Some will tell you why they have avoided treatment, but some will use other excuses for not going forward with care.

"Money" is the most common reason I hear patients give for not accepting treatment. As we explore this issue, it will become clear that money, or

---

14  Donaldson, Gizarelli, & Chanpong, "Oral Sedation: A Primer on Anxiolysis for the Adult Patient," 118.

the lack of it, is an important factor in patients' decision-making process but not to the degree most patients tell us. One of the easiest things for patients to do if they do not trust the dentist, are fearful, do not agree with treatment, or are not motivated is to tell the doctor the cost is too high for them.

Ask yourself this question: When someone is trying to sell you something, do you always give them the real reason when you say no? Have you ever said, "It's too much money" when prodded to buy? If friends suggest going away on vacation and you really do not want to spend a week away with them, is it easier to say, "I don't want to spend a week away with you" or "I don't want to (or can't) spend the money right now"?

When patients say they cannot afford treatment, it may be true. It is also just as possible that the patient has other reasons and finds it simply easier to avoid the uncomfortable truth.

I have often seen this to be the case with dental anxiety. I hear it in recordings of many appointments, but one in particular stood out. The dentist did a very good job of explaining the conditions and the options for treatment. He had a good connection with the patient, and throughout the appointment, the patient kept stressing that she could not afford it. She did not say it once or twice; literally five times during the appointment, she explained that she could not afford to do it right now.

Then, by chance, a strange thing happened. A discussion ensued about the difference between conventional and Cerec crowns. The patient explained that she was "irrationally fearful" about impressions. She was afraid she would choke. She then lowered her voice and whispered to the dentist, "If the truth were known, the money is really not such a big issue. I am just scared to death of impressions." When this issue was addressed to her satisfaction, she immediately chose treatment. However, it was purely an accident that the dentist found out she had a concern and money was not really the issue. The patient had done everything in her power up until that point to convince the dentist money was the problem. But what the dentist did well was to use the intangibles. He was not preoccupied but available and present with the patient, liked and appreciated her as a person, provided an environment that allowed her to hope for a better situation, and listened deeply to her view—and that allowed the patient to feel comfortable enough to reveal her true feelings.

As we discussed at the beginning of this section, this is not an isolated incident. Many, many patients have dental anxiety, and many will not tell you unless you ask and listen carefully. Once you know about the problem, whether you choose to use sedation dentistry as a tool or not, at least you can strategize how to support your patients in getting what they want and need.

## Agenda

*I don't apologize to people with an agenda.*

—KINKY FRIEDMAN

We discussed agendas earlier, but it's an important enough topic that we should explore it further and discuss a few more strategies. We all have agendas; it is just a question of what those agendas are. I have an agenda that you learn to communicate more effectively as a dental practitioner. If you have an agenda to learn new communications techniques, then we are in sync, and we can have a fruitful relationship. But if your agenda is to learn manipulative selling techniques, then you'll be seriously disappointed by this book. Your relationship and the way you interact with your patients are dictated by your agenda. So let's look a little deeper.

Though by no means a complete list, the following are some common agendas held by dentists:

- ❖ Help others
- ❖ Make money
- ❖ Perform specific procedures
- ❖ Avoid conflict
- ❖ Have control
- ❖ Have prestige
- ❖ Be liked
- ❖ Stay busy
- ❖ Avoid judgment

Some of these are in the conscious mind of the dentist, but many are not. You may know, for example, that you would like to try out a new technique you are interested in performing and that your next patient is the perfect candidate. You could have an agenda about wanting that patient to accept this specific treatment. This could be a slight desire on your part or it could be a strong desire or a need. On the other hand, you might not be as aware that you have an agenda to be liked by your patient and how that affects what you are willing to tell him.

For example, I have a client who stated that he does not like confrontation, and he began to realize that his agenda to avoid conflict was affecting his work. As happens in all practices, he had a difficult patient who had just had a lot of work done. The patient was pleased with the results, but in a follow-up visit, the dentist found a cavity and decided to hold off on telling the patient because he did not think the interaction would go well. His agenda to avoid conflict affected his quality of care. But by becoming aware of it, he could do something about it.

The dentist is only one side of the equation; another very important part is the agenda of the patient. As above, this list is by no means all inclusive, but the following are some common agendas held by patients (some of which may contribute to dental anxiety):

- ❖ Stay out of pain
- ❖ Avoid expense
- ❖ Be able to trust
- ❖ Be in control
- ❖ Be liked
- ❖ Avoid judgment
- ❖ Have a beautiful smile

As humans, in a lot of interactions, we negotiate. When it works, what we have is a meeting of agendas. Both people feel satisfied that what they want and need is being tended to sufficiently. Neither is simply "going along," and commitment is fostered instead of compliance.

Ideally it is best if dentists can leave their agendas at the door. So long as it does not violate what the dentist believes in and it is consistent with services the dentist wants to provide, the dentist should work toward understanding the patient and providing the patient with what he wants.

The absence of having an agenda is really what being present is all about. We are just there with the other person in the moment, meeting him where he is. When we go into our interactions with an agenda about the patient simply agreeing with us, it interferes with our ability to stay present and connected to him. But at times, having no agenda at all is difficult. All of us are human, and it may not always be possible to meet the patient with a blank canvas. You may want the patient to go forward with treatment because you would like the money. You may want the patient to go forward with treatment because you find it difficult to watch people lose teeth. So what do you do? Here are two approaches you might take.

First, if you cannot even temporarily leave your agenda at the door, at least acknowledge it. Tell the patient, "This is what I do for a living, and of course I would like to restore your teeth. However, what you want is what really matters, and it is more important that you want it than I."

In other words, make the agenda visible, and do not apologize for it, but also do not let it dictate what happens. Be authentic. All of us know at some level when the other person is not being authentic. When the auto mechanic says, "I really don't want to make three thousand dollars installing a new transmission," most of us find that a little difficult to believe. But when we get real with the other person and tell him, "Yes, I would like to see you do this, but it is up to you," a door opens and fresh air comes in. From this opening, patients can choose what is right for them. And often with this level of honesty, they learn to trust themselves and accept what you are saying, and from this place, they will choose a course that benefits everyone involved.

A second option is to consciously choose a more patient-focused agenda. Consciously replace the agenda that the patient says yes to treatment with the agenda to have a great connection with him. Since most of us are by nature goal oriented, change the goal. Make your goal to have a moment-by-moment, authentic, caring, and connected communication with the patient. Measure your success based on that agenda instead of whether the patient says yes. And of course, if you make having an authentic connection the focus, many patients will say yes.

## Commitment

*There's no abiding success without commitment.*

—TONY ROBBINS

There are only two fundamental ways patients move forward with treatment. They either do what they are told—they comply—or they understand, choose, and commit. A percentage of dentists are great at getting their patients to accept treatment. Most of the doctors I work with have stories about knowing a dentist like this. Their reputation is that if Dr. Williams goes into the room and tells the patient he needs it, he does it. I personally have met some of these doctors and have seen them in action, and there is no question it is true.

The problem is that these doctors generally get compliance and not commitment from their patients. They have such great presence, such dominant personalities and strong conviction about what they are proposing, that almost everyone says yes. Some of the patients who say yes basically trust they are getting what they need. Others are not sure about the need for treatment or why they need it. In some cases, the patient does not want the treatment being recommended but goes along with the doctor to avoid the confrontation.

Patients who comply and go forward with treatment present a number of problems for the dentist. These are the patients who go forward with treatment, but they accept it somewhat reluctantly. All trust has been placed in the doctor rather than the patient taking ownership of the decision for himself.

These are often the patients who resist paying their bills. Most people do not like spending money on needs-based dentistry. It is a little like paying taxes; it's a necessary evil. We like it even less when we do not fully understand it and did not fully choose it.

In addition, if the patient agrees to a root canal and the root canal fails, this type of patient is more likely to blame the doctor. It isn't something he really wanted in the first place. Now it is failing, and he has to do something else and pay more money. This same patient is also likely to be more annoyed by unexpected problems with treatment. If I really did not want a crown in the first place, I am more likely to be annoyed if the lab messes up and the crown needs to be remade.

A much better way to interact with a patient is to encourage commitment to treatment rather than compliance. Commitment comes when a patient first understands he has a problem and fully understands the consequences. This fosters a desire to learn the options for correcting and solving it.

From this place of understanding, the patient is actually generating the desire for treatment. He is doing it from a conscious place and is much more likely to be satisfied with the result than someone who is manipulated into treatment.

The other clear benefit to the doctor is that this approach requires a lot less effort on your part. A good sign that a patient is complying instead of committing is when you feel you are working harder at solving his problem than he is. When the patient is committed, the only work you do is the dentistry.

## Needs vs. Wants

Dentistry is somewhat unique in that most patients have dentistry they need and dentistry they want. At one time dentistry was almost solely about what one needed to do to keep teeth and maintain oral health. In fact, the current model for dentistry has grown out of, or was developed out of, this need-based model. However, especially since the advent of cosmetic dentistry, there are now patients who are interested in addressing elective wants. These wants can be a cosmetic smile or something as simple as a white composite filling instead of an amalgam.

Even within the group who are strictly concerned with their oral health, there is a wide range of options, values, and beliefs about what constitutes oral health. By addressing dental needs, patients are focused for the most part on avoiding a problem. Patients choose root canals to avoid losing a tooth. The mind-set of these patients, their attitude about choosing treatment, and their decision-making process could be compared to something like buying health insurance or life insurance. Treatment is chosen to avoid a problem or a more-serious consequence.

## Paint the Vision

*The only thing worse than being blind is having sight but no vision.*

—HELEN KELLER

In the case of cosmetic or wants-based dentistry, patients are excited about the benefits choosing treatment is likely to bring. This group may be more excited about that beautiful smile, asking about fixing gaps and straightening their teeth. This mind-set, attitude, and process is more like someone choosing to purchase a vacation. People choose it because they want it more than need it.

The point is that the way patients make decisions about wants-based dentistry and what they require from the dentist to make those decisions are very different than what they require to make a decision about choosing needs-based dentistry. Most dentists do not make the distinction in a conscious manner, and consequently they address both needs and wants in the same way. When it comes to wants-based dentistry it is important to paint a vision for patients about what is possible.

For example, Mr. Johnson enters your office for a comprehensive exam, and you notice he seems a bit hesitant to talk with you. He even seems a little embarrassed.

You ask him, "How are you doing today?"

He says, "OK I guess…"

"Just OK?"

"Fine; just a little old."

"Old?"

"Well, I'm turning fifty next week, and I'm feeling suddenly old."

"Ah, I turned fifty myself two years ago. I found it difficult too! Who thought I'd ever hit that day?"

"Tell me about it! I looked in the mirror, and I just can't believe the changes. I am my dad!"

"I understand. Well, we can't stop you from aging, but it's amazing how a few little changes in your teeth and smile can make you look much younger. If you're interested, when we go over your exam with you, I can give you some ideas about how the right teeth, color, and smile can take years off of your age."

"Well, yeah, that sounds great."

No one is likely to get sick or die from having an unattractive smile. However, a beautiful smile can go a long way toward creating great wedding photos or enhancing someone's self-esteem.

Much of modern dentistry is elective in nature, and patients do not always know what is available. In addition, even with needs-based dentistry, there are often choices regarding aesthetics that are important for the patient to understand when deciding on treatment options.

If communicating about needs-based dentistry is about creating awareness, explaining conditions and implications, and offering options, then wants-based dentistry is about painting the picture of what is possible. People make needs-based decisions based on how to avoid pain and problems. They make aesthetic decisions based on how it will make them feel and the benefits of looking good.

This type of interaction is more about how great the patient will look and feel. In following up on the conversation started at the beginning of this section with Mr. Johnson, during a Review of Findings Appointment, we might include in the patient's discussion the following.

"We can make you look younger by lengthening your upper teeth and whitening. From what you have told me, you will be thrilled you did it."

"How will that help?"

"One of the diagnostic factors in gauging how youthful your smile is concerns how much upper tooth you display when your lips are relaxed. As you can see, in this picture of your lip at rest, we don't see your upper teeth at all, and in fact see quite a bit of your lower teeth. This is due to a number of things. As we get older, the muscles around our mouths change shape and tone, thereby changing the shape and tone of our lips and mouth. By lengthening your upper teeth and adding a little bulk, we will fill out those parts of your face that have shifted over time, smoothing wrinkles and giving you a more youthful appearance. Let me show you some before-and-after pictures."

Clearly this kind of conversation is different than talking to patients about losing their teeth. But by listening to them and painting the vision of a brighter dental future, you support them in building hope. From this place, they are more likely to say yes to wants-based procedures.

## Reinforce Treatment Decisions

*I like to encourage people to realize that any action is a good action if it's proactive and there is positive intent behind it.*

—MICHAEL J. FOX

All of us want to feel good about the decisions we make. After you've performed treatment on a patient, it is important to reinforce the patient's decision to go forward with treatment.

I have met some dentists who are great at supporting patients in their decision to go forward with treatment. From the time patients make the decision to completion of the work, these dentists make a point of telling them, "I think you made a great decision that supports the goals you want." As I mentioned earlier, this isn't meant as false praise. If you don't feel the patient made a good decision, don't say you do. But if you've been present, listened to the patient, and can appreciate him for what he had to go through to make the decision he did, even if it doesn't completely agree with what you feel is the best dental decision, you'll likely see it was a great decision for him at this time. And if you can get to that place of understanding, why not say it to him? It's another way for you and the patient to continue to build a relationship.

In addition, often during treatment, these dentists will take photographs while preparing the teeth, showing any decay or needs-based work and explaining why it was good that the patients took care of the issues. This continues the process of letting patients know what is happening in their mouths. After treatment, dentists will tell these patients how good the changes look and have staff members and other doctors come in to reinforce the impression. They do this even though the patients have already said yes and are going forward with treatment.

From before treatment to a year later in a hygiene-recall appointment, it is helpful to remind wants-based patients of their healthy and wise decision. I suspect it goes a long way toward encouraging the patients to choose future treatment and to refer their friends.

Now that we've discussed how to communicate with patients, in chapter 4, we'll look at how we as health care practitioners trip ourselves up. Our past learning often leaves us with a belief that we need to take care of our patients because they can't take care of themselves. We'll explore how dangerous and counterproductive this belief is—to both you and your patients—and give you a few more methods to build healthy relationships with them.

## Summary of Key Points

❖ *Why Not Decide for the Patient?* The patient who does not accept treatment is as, if not more, important than the one who does.

❖ *Awareness Is the Foundation of Change.* Our job is to create awareness. The patient's job is to act on that awareness.

❖ *Trust.* Trust is a function of the clinician's integrity and the patient fully understanding his or her choices.

❖ *Keep it Simple.* Speak plainly, and use visuals, analogies, and metaphors.

❖ *Needs vs. Wants.* With needs, communicate the implications of the conditions. With wants, focus on what is possible.

❖ *Your Patient Knows.* The first step in helping your patients is in understanding their goals.

# CHAPTER 4

# Caretaking and Money

## Caretaking vs. Compassion

*The purpose of human life is to serve, and to show compassion and the will to help others.*

—ALBERT SCHWEITZER

It is Saturday night, and you're ready to go out for a meal. Maybe your mouth is already watering for that first bite. You ask your spouse or partner, "Where would you like to go for dinner?"

He or she responds, "I don't care. What would you like to do?"

You think about it for a moment, and you're in the mood for an informal, easy burger and a beer at the new café down the street. But you think your significant other really likes that upscale Italian restaurant, and you're not sure he or she is being completely honest with you about not caring where you go. Besides, you really don't want to deal with his or her unspoken disappointment should you choose something unwanted. So you respond by asking, "How about that Italian restaurant?"

If you have ever had an experience like this, you at some level understand the basic concept of caretaking versus caregiving. Simply put:

*Caretaking occurs when I modify my behavior because I do not want to experience your reaction.*

In this example, one person modifies his behavior by ultimately assuming what the other person wants to do without speaking his own want—not out of caring but out of not wanting to experience her rejection, anger, or whatever would cause him discomfort if experienced.

The flip side of caretaking is caregiving, in which we do something for another person not because of a concern for his reaction but rather genuinely from our hearts. For example, most parents can relate to doing something for their children simply because they want to do so. One of the ways to know the difference between the two is asking yourself the questions, "Would I do this even if I knew the other person wouldn't react negatively?" or "Would I do this even if knew no one would ever know I did it?"

Often people find these two concepts—caregiving and caretaking—confusing. They're not sure which is happening when. This confusion is natural and occurs because they both have a similar root; both typically come from an origin of compassion and caring. The same behavior could be observed from the outside as looking very similar, but it's really where it comes from. One stays pure and clean, and the other becomes defensive in nature.

Caregiving in the dinner example would be asking the question because you genuinely want to give your spouse or partner what he or she wants rather than being fearful of the reaction that might come back at you. It is a simple concept, but it is pervasive in our culture and most cultures. It has serious implications for all relationships and certainly for dentists who are attempting to communicate comprehensive-care dentistry or simply to connect with their patients.

Take, for example, the situation in which a dentist is preparing to talk about a possible treatment plan with a patient where she is concerned the patient is likely to be angry about the cost. Maybe she has seen this patient get angry before around discussions involving money. Or maybe she has her own limiting beliefs about money and simply expects the patient to be angry. For the moment, regardless of the dentist's reasons, let's operate from the premise that she is anxious about the patient getting angry. How will this anxiety impact what she says to the patient and the way she says it? Maybe the dentist will avoid the money discussion by passing it on to someone else, like the office manager. Maybe she will be defensive or angry to preempt the patient's anger. Or possibly she will jump to solutions, such as phasing treatment or presenting less-than-optimal care as a way to avoid conflict before even exploring what is best for the patient.

Caretaking is not always about money or anger, but in general, it has four major components:

1) the trigger (in this case money);
2) the anticipated reaction from the patient that we do not want to experience;
3) how that anticipated reaction makes us feel; and
4) the behavior or defense we choose in order to avoid the anticipated reaction and subsequent feelings.

Instead of money, we could use patient fear. The reaction we do not want to experience could be tears, the feeling we want to avoid could be sadness, and the behavior we use to avoid those feelings could be to tell the patient he "shouldn't be feeling anything."

The *trigger* can be anything about which the dentist is concerned the patient will have an emotional reaction. This can be because of some knowledge about the patient or because the dentist has a history involving this particular trigger.

The *anticipated patient reaction* is how the patient might respond to the situation, and it's really what we *believe* will happen versus what is *actually* happening. This dialogue with ourselves occurs before the patient is even aware of the topic! This anticipation makes the dentist feel uncomfortable.

*How the anticipated patient reaction makes us feel* is the uncomfortable feelings we experience and want to avoid. The avoided feelings can be completely different than what the dentist anticipates the patient will feel. For example, a dentist may be afraid of feeling fear generated by the patient exhibiting anger. Often, however, the avoided feelings are the same or similar to the anticipated patient's reaction. For example, the patient feels fearful and that triggers or reminds the dentist of her own feelings of fear.

Finally, in an effort to avoid these uncomfortable feelings, the dentist may protect himself by using a *defense* or protection. For example, to avoid feelings of being rejected, the dentist may resort to pleasing the patient by refraining from giving uncomfortable news. Table 1 provides several scenarios of caretaking and how it's played out.

Table 1 Components and Examples of Caretaking

| Common Triggers | Anticipated Patient Reaction | Dentist's Avoided Feelings | Dentist's Defense |
|---|---|---|---|
| Money | ➡ Anger | ➡ Fear | ➡ Withdrawal |
| Pain | Fear | Sadness | Judgment |
| Embarrassment | Sadness | Sadness | Pleasing |
| Uncomfortable News | Judgment | Abandonment | Rejection |

## THE WAY OF THE SUPERIOR DENTIST

As we delve into this concept a little deeper, we find it happens in a lot of places in our lives and the lives of our patients. Unfortunately, the impact is to undermine the relationship we have been striving to create because both the dentist and the patient find themselves in a defensive/protective stance. The trust is eroded, and real communication becomes impossible. To better understand how to deal with caretaking, it is useful to explore why we do it in the first place.

As with most behaviors, we learn caretaking at a very early age. When we are born, we are completely dependent for our survival on others. Most of the time, this dependency is upon our primary caregivers, and in most cases, that's our parents. In our earliest years, this dependence is greatest. As we grow older, we become less physically dependent, but we are not fully aware that our survival is no longer at stake. Usually we consciously realize we are not that vulnerable child, but unconsciously we often still have that feeling or belief that we are dependent.

As human beings, we begin our journey in the world literally as a part of our mother's body. What happens to our mother during pregnancy is actually happening to us as well. There is no distinction between self and other.

After birth for quite some time, we still have no ability to separate who we are from others around us. From this way of looking at the world, we begin to see ourselves as responsible for what is happening to others.

Take the example of a small child who claps his hands and his mom laughs and congratulates him. The child believes he is causing the parent's happiness. He does not understand that the parent has her own experience; the child believes it is all in his power. The same holds true if the parent becomes angry at the child; the child also believes he has the power to cause his mom's anger and modifies his behavior to keep that from happening again. It is not unusual for a parent to say something to a child like, "Stop crying; you are driving me crazy!" The child already thinks he's the center of the universe and all that happens, and this reinforces the belief by telling him he has the power to determine the parent's emotions. It's based in survival and makes sense for that young child, but it begins a pattern that carries forward in the child's life.

As we grow older, if we have the right environment, we begin to make the distinction between self and other. However, many of us still carry forward those early beliefs, unconsciously still thinking that we are responsible for other people's feelings and behaviors.

In addition to our inherent belief that we are responsible for others, another important contributor to caretaking is our concern that feelings will overwhelm us. When we are young, we are more vulnerable to these feelings than when we are adults. Yelling and screaming have much more of an impact on a young child than a full-grown adult. When these strong feelings come when we are children, we need to find a way to cope with them. We might avoid, get angry, or try to please people to keep from experiencing these intense emotions. The problem for many of us is that we developed the belief at a very young age that these strong feelings are intolerable. As we grow, we get stuck in the past and come to believe these feelings will be too much for us and for others, even as adults. To protect ourselves from this imaginary danger, we use avoidant behavior, also called defenses.

Although defenses typically have a negative connotation, as children they were often necessary for our emotional survival, and as adults they can have their time and place. Some of the more-destructive defenses include things like drinking, gambling, and other addictions. For our purposes, we will focus on some of the less outwardly destructive defenses, such as withdrawal, pleasing, avoidance, judgment, rejection, arrogance, and other similar ways of protecting ourselves. And although they are certainly preferable to the more-destructive defenses, we still pay a high price for using them, and they definitely impact our relationships with our patients.

Children learn most defenses from their parents. If I see my mother pleasing my father to keep him out of a certain mood, it is not unusual for me to learn to do the same thing. If you look closely at your defenses (and we all have them), you will probably see you learned them at a very early age.

These defenses are utilized to caretake *ourselves* from experiencing emotional reactions we are trying to avoid. Most of us, if we recognize we are caretaking, tell ourselves we are doing it to be nice to the other person, and I suspect that often there is an element of genuine compassion or caring in the caretaking. But most caretaking is of a defensive nature. Let's look at another example of where we learn this caretaking behavior.

Imagine a five-year-old watching her mother crying because she has just had a fight with her husband. Watching the person she depends on for her survival in pain is difficult. It is also not completely clear to the five-year-old that this is not happening to her or that she is not somehow responsible. She goes to her mother and brings her a picture she drew at school to make her feel better. Her mother responds positively and gives her a hug, and the little girl feels better; she believes she has the ability to take care and change her mother's feelings. Her mother, in her pain, may even say something to the little girl like, "I don't know what I would do without you."

The little girl believes she has succeeded in getting her mother to act and feel differently. But what happened to the little girl's feelings? How was she feeling watching her mother cry? Was she afraid, confused, hurt? Her feelings do not get expressed, but she has protected herself from them by doing something she believes has gotten her mother to stop crying. This defense was smart and necessary as a child. But over time, the girl keeps using these methods of managing the distress of her parents, and eventually, as an adult, she uses this defense in many feelings of discomfort—with her spouse, her boss, and even her own children, passing on this coping mechanism to the next generation. And through it all, those original feelings of fear, confusion, and pain sit below the surface, untended, guiding these unconscious reactions and keeping her from experiencing the fullness of relationships that come from honest, expressed emotions.

And there's another important point here—the girl did not actually make the mother act differently. She did not have that power. The little girl did take an action her mother liked, but it was her mother who chose to change her behavior. This distinction may seem like a small one, but it's important to understand: the child never actually had the power to change her mother's feelings or behaviors, just like we don't have the power as adults to change another's behavior. We are not really the center of the universe, and we can let ourselves off the hook of that burden.

Let's take a look at another common version of caretaking alluded to above: the act of denying another person's experience. This one often occurs in healthcare. How many times is a patient told, "You're not in pain; I gave you plenty of anesthesia." Now this may sound crazy, and it is, but it happens all the time. Why do we do it? I think it's because we are uncomfortable that the patient is uncomfortable, or because if we cannot alleviate the patient's pain, we feel incompetent. It is not unusual for patients to sense your need for them to be comfortable, and they may caretake your feelings by telling you they are doing OK when they are not.

Ultimately caretaking is when I take responsibility for your feelings. Oftentimes I decide for you how you are feeling about something whether it is true or not. For example, let's assume I begin a conversation with you about your dental condition. I look over at you, and your mouth is turned down. I decide you are upset with me for giving you this bad news. Without checking with you, because I do not want you to be upset (because I do not want to experience your reaction or because I experience your disappointment or upset as though it is happening to me), I immediately jump to telling you we have other alternatives.

There are a lot of assumptions here.

## THE WAY OF THE SUPERIOR DENTIST

First, I am assuming you are upset, and I could easily be wrong. I remember once talking to colleague who would get a certain look on her face. I would think she was upset. After talking to her, she explained to me that when she got that particular look, it meant she was concentrating, not upset. We rarely accurately assess people's internal meaning by their external demeanor.

Second, if I am right about how you are feeling, I may or may not be right about *why* you are feeling that way. You might have had a terrible day before seeing me, and your mind may have gone to those thoughts during our conversation—and I'm suddenly changing treatment plans based on this assumption.

Last, I believe that by changing my behavior, I will change your feeling. Given that I don't really know what you're feeling or why you're feeling it, how I act can have little bearing on what's truly happening and can often make the situation even more confusing.

The message we are really giving the people in our lives is that it is not OK for them to feel how they feel. Even if we are right about all of our assumptions about how they are feeling and the reasons, we are trying to take away their right to feel that way.

How do you feel when you are angry at someone and then the person agrees to do what you want, and you believe it is because he or she does not want you to be angry? I know that personally, it does not feel good for me to think people modified their behavior to keep me from being angry. I also get the message that it is not OK to feel or express my anger.

For the people doing the caretaking, there is some relief that the person is not angry, but there is also a sense of giving themselves away, and in effect, denying their own needs to accommodate the other person. As stated above, but important to reiterate: though I may take an action and the other person may change his behavior, I did not make him change. I don't have that power. He chose to change what he was doing based on what he was observing.

I believe the greatest negative to caretaking is the loss of emotional intimacy that results. Caretaking (especially the pleasing version) often appears to be selfless. The person doing the caretaking appears to be a person who just does things for other people out of the goodness of his heart. He's such a nice guy, he would give you the shirt off of his back, he is always saying nice things, he is so considerate, so sweet etc.... Everyone knows someone like this.

Is this really selfless? I suppose it is possible, but I have not seen it. More often than not it is really to protect the person engaging in the caretaking. She does not want the other person to be angry with her, or she wants to be liked and avoid being told she is not nice. Or maybe she finds it very uncomfortable to be in the presence of another person's discomfort for the reasons mentioned earlier. In any of these cases, who is really the focus of the caretaking? The person doing the caretaking! We are really not doing it from a place of caring about the other person but rather as a self-protection. My experience is that *caretaking is a very self-centered behavior.* This is not a surprise because it is a child behavior, and children are by nature ego centric or self-centered.

When is doing something for someone caretaking, and when is it compassionate caregiving? Caretaking has the agenda of protecting oneself from feeling bad or guilty or experiencing an unpleasant emotion or behavior. There may be genuine caring for the other person, but the caretaking is driven by things like wanting to be liked.

Compassion, on the other hand, is just allowing the other person to be where she is and letting her heart touch your heart without any need to fix her pain. One can care about another without trying to fix or change her feelings.

So what can we do about our tendency to caretake a patient's feelings? The most helpful thing we can do is to heal the part of us that is uncomfortable feeling the avoided feelings. We can do this through some form of counseling, therapy, and in some cases, self-reflection. We revisit those places in our past where we learned the behavior, and with compassion, we can retrain ourselves to no longer have that defensive reaction.

Although this retraining is the ideal solution, it is not always possible to catch and heal what needs to be healed in the moment when the feelings are happening. In this case, the second-best option is to become self-aware of these feelings and catch ourselves moving toward caretaking and consciously take a different tack. For example, if you notice a patient beginning to get angry, you notice your reaction of fear and remind yourself that although the fear you are feeling was appropriate as a child, you are now safe, and you can make a conscious decision not to act from a place of caretaking now. This is often easier said than done, but you will find that with a little practice, you can manage your internal feelings (see the "Going Deeper" section of this chapter for ways to practice).

Finally, if you find yourself triggered beyond your ability to respond from a non-caretaking stance, you may find taking a break from the conversation and coming back to it when you feel stronger a better way to deal with more-difficult situations.

Most of us have spent at least a portion of our lives practicing ways of being that don't support us, and those old patterns can be deeply ingrained. But mastering your tendency to caretake is of critical importance in creating authentic, connected relationships with your patients. We can learn again to build a new habit that allows the patients their feelings and in the end, can build better relationships with the people sitting in our chairs.

## Going Deeper

*Pausing is very helpful in this process. It creates a momentary contrast between being completely self-absorbed and being awake and present. You just stop for a few seconds, breathe deeply, and move on. You don't want to make it into a project... You pause and allow there to be a gap in whatever you're doing.*

—PEMA CHODRON, TAKING THE LEAP

Imagine for a moment that you are stressed out. This could be for any reason that comes to you in the moment—whether it's something that happens for you at home, with anticipation of what will happen with a patient, or financial reasons, you feel you're under more stress than normal. From the following list, pick three items you'd be most likely to do:

- ❖ *Withdraw*

- ❖ *Use humor*

- ❖ *Change the subject*

- ❖ *Avoid by doing something else*—sleep, run/exercise, sex, go to a movie, etc.

- ❖ *Please others*

- ❖ *Stop the feelings*—via chemicals, alcohol, or some other method

- ❖ *Reject*

- ❖ *Get angry*

- ❖ *Get depressed*

- ❖ *Stay in self-pity*

- ❖ *Freeze*

- ❖ *Blame it on others*

- ❖ *Get people around me upset* and look for validation on how bad it is

These are probably your primary defenses and are probably things you learned a very long time ago. Growing up, you probably did these most often in some form or fashion, and you may have learned them by watching your parents do them. When you're in these defenses and not in the true you, it's helpful to build awareness so you can come back out of them. Defenses are normal, but the problem comes when they are unconscious, and you're simply on autopilot. The most helpful thing in the moment is to just bring mindfulness and awareness. Start to realize when you've withdrawn—notice when you become angry and bring self-awareness, and you'll have more control over your defenses. Take baby steps first. The first step is awareness alone.

Begin to practice pausing in your life. Put a picture in a place you see many times a day, and whenever you see that picture, stop for a moment and come back to you. Or set an alarm on your phone that plays a pleasing tone every so often, and when you hear that tone, take a deep breath. Just one breath. If, as Pema Chodron states above, you can create a small gap between a triggering moment and tromping unconsciously down the path of one of your defenses, you've become more aware, and you've stepped out of the realm of reaction and into the realm of choice.

## Money

*The love of money is the root of all evil.*

—1 TIMOTHY 6:10 KJV

*A penny saved is a penny earned.*

—BENJAMIN FRANKLIN

*He has more money than God.*

*She's filthy rich.*

*Time is money.*

—BENJAMIN FRANKLIN

*A fool and his money are easily parted.*

—THOMAS TUSSER

*Too many of us look upon Americans as dollar chasers. This is a cruel libel, even if it is reiterated thoughtlessly by the Americans themselves.*

—ALBERT EINSTEIN

Few things throw dentists off their center as easily as the issue of money. When it comes to the Emotional Exam, Clinical Exam or Review of Findings appointment, the dentist can be going along without any struggle discussing conditions, implications, and solutions, the whole time focused on the patient and how best to serve him. Then along comes a concern, or even a simple question or statement about money or the cost of treatment, and the doctor loses the ability to serve the patient from a place of clarity.

I have heard more than one Review of Findings appointment where the patient expresses a concern about cost, and the dentist literally ignores the comment or question and continues the review of the patient's mouth. As mentioned earlier, in one, the patient brought up his concerns about being able to afford treatment *five different times*, and each time, the doctor either paused and changed the subject or talked over him.

Other responses I hear include arguing with the patient that either the dentist or the treatment is worth it or moving straight to financing options. What I hear most often, though, is an uncomfortable, partial acknowledgment of the financial issues and a hand-off to a front desk person or patient coordinator to discuss these unpleasant details.

How is it that a dentist, with all of her training and skill and the ability to both manage a staff and handle serious medical emergencies, can be so thrown off by simple questions and comments about money? Dentists are not alone when it comes to having difficulties with this subject. In our society, much is wrapped up in the concept of charging, earning, paying, having, deserving, and accumulating money.

I often joke with my clients that they are more likely to tell me how many times they had sex last week than they are to tell me how much money they have in the bank or how much debt they have! There is so much confusion and shame in our society about money that it is no surprise doctors and patients struggle around this issue of the cost of the patient's treatment.

As we explore what makes money such a problem for the health care provider, it is useful to keep in mind that patients are carrying their own dysfunctional views about money. The beliefs and meaning surrounding money are very complex. From the quotes at the beginning of this section, look at some of the powerful and conflicting messages our society has been exposed to and in many cases absorbed.

I suspect given the time, most readers could add to that list. Money is a highly charged subject, and the subconscious beliefs we have absorbed for the most part come from our childhood. I highly recommend that anyone who has anything to do with money (all of us), but especially dentists who deal with this every day, explore their subconscious beliefs about money and make them conscious.

There are some great resources available to do just that. One suggestion is to read the book *The Energy of Money* by Maria Nemeth, a clinical psychologist who once lost thirty-five thousand dollars in an investment scam, chose to investigate why, and developed a workshop and book to support others in their process.

## Dentistry vs. General Medicine

I suggest dentists especially investigate their beliefs because when it comes to money, they are in a unique situation compared to most other traditional health care providers. The traditional model for health care is the insurance model that, in general, pays for treatment the doctor determines is necessary. If you go to your primary care physician and he or she determines you need a particular test, in most cases it is paid for in full or with a small co-payment.

If you have a life-threatening illness, in most situations your insurance will pay for most of the treatment necessary. [15]

As you know, in the dental world the use of the term *dental insurance* is inaccurate. Dental insurance is really a benefit, usually paid for by the patient's employer, that covers a specific amount of care each year. Further, the dental benefit makes a distinction between what is needs-based dentistry and what is deemed cosmetic (or wants-based) dentistry.

The idea that some dentistry is needs based and some is wants based makes it somewhat unique. For the most part, your primary care physician is interested in prevention and needs-based health care. If you focus on wants-based services, you visit a different doctor, perhaps your local plastic surgeon.

But dentists are different; they deal with both ends of the spectrum. There is certainly a part of dentistry that is about patient health. Periodontal disease or an abscessed tooth has direct impact on the patient's health. At the other end of the spectrum, veneers for the sole purpose of cosmetics are wants-based dentistry. To complicate matters more, there are many procedures that fall somewhere in the middle. Replacing a missing tooth in an older person has some health benefits and some cosmetic benefits.

It is this combination of needs/wants care and the insurance benefit model that make working with money very different in dentistry than in general medicine.

---

15   This is not to say this system is not fraught with problems. It definitely is, and we hear about it daily on the news as there are more and more conversations about universal health care and our health care system in general. On several occasions I have had the opportunity to consult with physicians, and I'm stunned by how hard most of them work for a lot less than most people realize. If you look at physicians compared to dentists, the majority of dentists I work with come out way ahead, especially when you factor in the cost for training and the hours worked by each. This was not always true. There was a time when physicians made significantly more money than the average dentist, but that has changed as general medicine has moved in the direction of HMOs.

In addition, how dentists approach their patients has a great effect on how they handle money with them. Whether you caretake or caregive greatly influences how you approach money topics and patient care. They are interwoven.

## Strategies for Dealing with Money

When we combine the complicated beliefs most people hold around money with the human tendency for caretaking, it is no surprise that money is such a difficult issue for many of us. Fully dealing with money and caretaking is beyond the scope of this book, but my hope is that awareness of the problem and a few suggestions may be helpful and start you on a new path.

First I would encourage you to explore and make yourself as conscious as possible about your beliefs concerning money. Whether you take a workshop, read a book, or talk about it with staff and friends, really come to know what your beliefs about money are and how they impact you. One way to do that is to just talk about money and where you learned what you learned. How did your father deal with money, and how did your mother? Was it out in the open? Do you remember the first time you earned money? How did it feel?

Questions like these can be a powerful way to explore your memories and beliefs about money. As you do that, they become conscious and you gain some control over what is often a knee-jerk reaction to the triggers of money. I highly recommend that you try the going deeper exercises at the end of this section.

## Setting Fees

Another problem I encounter is dentists having fees that do not reflect their values. Often dentists set their fees based on wanting to get ego satisfaction from the fee. All of the best prosthodontists in the area are charging twenty-six hundred dollars for a crown, so the dentist sets her fee at twenty-six hundred dollars. The story she tells herself is that if she charges less, the patient will not believe she is any good. Or maybe she believes she will satisfy an internal need to feel good about herself by the patients saying yes to the fee.

The problem is that if dentists do not feel a strong conviction about how the service they are providing justifies the fee they are charging, they feel it and in turn the staff and patients feel it. Sometimes this discomfort takes the form of avoiding fee discussions or a defensiveness about the fee.

I suggest setting your fees at or just slightly below what you feel is fair. I know this is contrary to some of the conventional wisdom. Some will tell you to set the fee higher and feel good about it. If you really can do that, I agree—a little stretch that is within the market rate is something you can see as a challenge but not an overwhelming challenge. But if you think it is going to impact your ability to talk confidently to a patient about fees, I would not do it. Instead, I would suggest starting out a little on the lower side, and as you gain confidence and get acceptance from patients, you can slowly raise your fee. It is important to keep in mind that the reason for setting your fee a little lower is not because the patient will care, but it will make a difference for you and how you communicate. Patients will generally feel that dentistry is expensive; whether you charge twelve hundred dollars or eighteen hundred dollars for that crown, it will seem like a lot for many people. What will be different, however, is if you feel twelve hundred dollars is low, you will communicate it like it is a bargain. If eighteen hundred dollars is high in your area, you will most likely communicate it with a defensiveness or lack of confidence.

## Be Real

*Soul is about authenticity*

—JOHN LEGEND

Once you have an awareness of any beliefs or defenses regarding money and you have set your fees at a level that you feel are fair, then it is about being real. When a patient asks questions about finances, answer them. Handle these questions directly and honestly. In many offices it works best to have a person from the front or a treatment coordinator to discuss the specifics of financial arrangements with the patient. However, this should not be a substitute for the dentist answering and addressing questions the patient may ask. If a patient asks, "How much is all of this going to cost?" I do not suggest responding with, "I will go over the dentistry, and Mary, our treatment coordinator, will discuss finances." This is a mistake for two reasons. First and most important, the patient will feel you are avoiding something (and you probably are). The second is that the treatment needs to be in alignment with the patient's objectives. If the cost does not work, it needs to be addressed. This does not always mean changing the treatment plan, but it does need to be acknowledged.

Simply say to the patient, "If we do everything we have talked about, the cost will be between twenty-five thousand dollars and thirty thousand dollars. I do not know precisely, but our treatment coordinator Mary can give you more exact numbers. Does this work for your budget?"

The exact wording is not important, but what is important is to answer honestly and directly and invite the patient to tell you whether that works for him. If you feel good about the treatment, good about your fees, and are not feeling a need to caretake the patient, this becomes an easy conversation. And because you are being direct and honest and have been tailoring your recommendations to the patient's objectives, most patients will not have a strong reaction.

If the patient does have a strong reaction, take it head on. Let's assume for a moment the patient says something like, "You must be crazy. I'm not going to spend thirty thousand dollars on my teeth."

I would suggest responding like this: "It sounds like I caught you by surprise. I am sorry about that." Pause. Let the patient absorb that and respond.

Oftentimes a simple pause is enough for the patient to come up with his own solution. If not, then you might continue by saying something like, "I understood that you did not want to lose your teeth. I can hear now that you did not realize what it will cost to do that. There are less-expensive options, but there are some consequences. The other options will most likely result in losing most if not all of the teeth we talked about."

Notice that there is not any defensiveness on the part of the doctor. The doctor does not apologize for the cost itself but does acknowledge in the communication that maybe the way the cost was communicated caught the patient off guard. The doctor then brings the patient back to his objectives and points out the conflict. It is now up to the patient to help the doctor know what to do next. The patient may clarify and reconsider the cost, in which case it may be appropriate to talk about phasing treatment or financing options. I do not suggest talking about phasing treatment and financing options until the patient has told you he would like to do the dentistry if the finances could be made to work. This mistake is common in many offices. Utilizing financing as a way to get case acceptance before the patient is committed to treatment is typically received as a form of manipulation, not unlike the car salesman who asks, "What will it take for you buy this car today?"

## Going Forward

Money and caretaking are deep issues that are informed by our upbringing, experience, and learned behaviors. Awareness of your underlying beliefs is extremely important to successfully building a relationship with your patients. Caretaking may be the number-one impediment to communicating with patients, but money is a close second. Changing these beliefs and behaviors takes time and self-reflection, and it's important to recognize that no technique will work without it coming from a clear place. And no clear place is possible without significant self-reflection and exploration.

## Going Deeper

Working with your beliefs around money takes time and courage. To start you off, try these exercises. I encourage you to write your answers so you can go back and review your thoughts over time.

1) Take a ten-dollar bill and tear it up into pieces that are smaller than a quarter of the bill. Now write about what comes up for you. Did you feel anxious? Angry? Frightened? Trace that feeling back to when you first felt it in your life. What was happening then? How old were you? Now, imagine if you ripped up a twenty-dollar bill or a hundred-dollar bill. Would your feelings change? How so?

2) Taking the exercise above, how would your parents feel or have felt about you ripping up money? What would they have told you? What were your parents' beliefs? Were they frightened of money? Did they live as if they never had enough? Or did they have so much it didn't matter? How did those beliefs affect you? How did they inform your beliefs?

3) Find a quiet time and a place where you will have some privacy. Using either a journal or a computer, sit and write your money story. Take the time to write about your earliest memories of earning money, spending money, and hearing your parents talk about money. Be as detailed as possible, and write with as little judgment as possible. The goal here is to make conscious all of the many memories you have about money. Write this as though no one else will ever read it. I recommend writing for at least thirty minutes.

## Summary of Key Points

- *Caretaking.* Caretaking occurs when I modify my behavior because I do not want to experience your reaction. It undermines the relationship we have been striving to create because both the dentist and the patient find themselves in a defensive/protective stance. Trust is eroded, and real communication becomes impossible. In caregiving, we do something for another person not because of a concern for his or her reaction but rather genuinely from our heart.

- *Money.* Know your own beliefs about money, and recognize that your patients and your team also have beliefs about money that impact their actions and decisions.

# PART 2:

# A Step-by-Step Guide

**CHAPTER 5**

# Components of Relationship-Centered Dentistry

*I'm not an amazing cook. But I can follow a recipe!*

—RACHEL MCADAMS

Part 2 of this book will take you through creating the basic structure you will use to develop a relationship-centered practice. In general, this process involves communicating comprehensive-care dentistry through every phase and by every member of your staff while in the course of treating a patient. But more importantly, it is a way of building a relationship and partnering with your patients such that you provide them a complete view and options for optimal dental health based on their needs and desires.

## Classic Dental Practices

In a typical practice, offices use the New Patient Clinical Exam, some form of Periodic or Hygiene Exam, and an Emergency Exam to interact with patients. During the New Patient Exam, the patient receives radiographs, a periodontal exam, and a tooth charting. During or at the end of that same appointment, treatment needs are discussed and recommended.

During a Periodic Exam or Hygiene Check, patients are often examined in a similar but shortened version of the New Patient Exam. In some practices, this is the only time treatment is recommended. In an Emergency Exam, the patient receives care for the emergency and is often told about other treatment recommendations at the same time.

Although these exams can vary from office to office, this represents what we see most often. In the following we will offer a different approach to communicating, diagnosing, and recommending treatment to patients.

## Relationship Centered Practice

With the relationship-centered approach, we tend to place more emphasis on the human being than is seen in exams in the typical dental practice. The tools for this approach are outlined in the box to the right. As we dive deeper into the practical aspects of delivering relationship-centered/comprehensive-care dentistry, it will help to define the different types of dental exams,

**Elements of the Relationship Centered Approach**

- Emotional Exam ⎫
- Clinical Exam ⎪
- Photographs ⎬ Comprehensive Exam
- Review of Findings Appointment ⎪
- Hygiene/Emergency Exams ⎭

both in terms of how they are typically used and how that contrasts with the way they will be used when creating a relationship-centered practice.

- ❖ The *Comprehensive Exam* is made up of four parts: the Emotional and Clinical Exams, Photographs, and Review of Findings Appointment.
    - o The *Emotional Exam* allows you to know the person behind the teeth. It is more about listening and understanding patients' goals, hopes, fears, attitudes, beliefs, approaches, and behaviors that impact their dental health and health in general. Although you will hopefully learn about the patient's dental condition, it is not the primary purpose of this appointment. It's important for you to be mindful of and bring in the skills of all four intangibles discussed in part 1. The Emotional Exam probably requires the most attention to learn because it is different than what most dentists are trained to do. But once mastered, it is an invaluable tool in creating a relationship-centered dental practice.
    - o The *Clinical Exam* follows the Emotional Exam and is most like New Patient Exams found in typical practices. The greatest difference here is that rather than examining the patient and giving her the dentist's findings, the dentist involves the patient in the exam.
    - o *Photographs.* During the Clinical Exam, you'll take intraoral photographs that will help you during, and act as the tie to, the Review of Findings Appointment. These photographs are an important step to showing the patient your findings and collaborating with her for treatment.
    - o The *Review of Findings (ROF) Appointment* generally occurs one to two weeks after the Comprehensive Exam and is similar to what many practices call a case presentation. The major difference between the typical case presentation and a Review of Findings Appointment is that this appointment is less about presenting and more about reviewing what was discovered by you and the

patient during the Emotional Exam and Clinical Exam and together, confirming potential treatment options.
- ❖ You'll then use the *Hygiene* and *Emergency Exams* to support the entire process.

Let's dive into the process at the beginning with preparing for the Comprehensive Exam.

## Setting the Table

Approach your Comprehensive Exam appointments in the same way you approach getting ready for any other appointment or procedure. If you are planning on performing a crown preparation, you start by having an operatory to work in, functioning equipment, enough time, an assistant, and the proper materials. Of course, sometimes you are not able to work under ideal conditions, but you do not intentionally plan to prepare a crown in the hygiene operatory without an assistant in thirty minutes and without the materials.

When it comes to communicating treatment, it is often done on the fly, without the planning, support, and necessary tools. However, any preparation you make for this appointment will pay large dividends.

## Consult Room

It is important to have the right environment in which to meet with the patient. For the Emotional Exam and the Review of Findings Appointment, ideally they should not be in the operatory. An operatory has everything necessary to perform examinations and dental procedures, but it is not the ideal place to comfortably meet with the patient. In some offices, there is no other place to conduct the Emotional Exam or Review of Findings appointment, but if at all possible, even if it is just a quiet part of the office, I recommend using that space. If you are fortunate and have a room you can dedicate for this purpose, or maybe one that doubles for another purpose, that is best. (Note: If you must use the operatory for these nonclinical appointments, have the patient sit upright in a chair other than the dental chair.)

Instead of a clinical room, create the look and feel of a consult room. Clear out as much clutter as possible, and make it relaxed and comfortable. It is not important for it to look fancy or expensive, but it should be a relaxing environment.

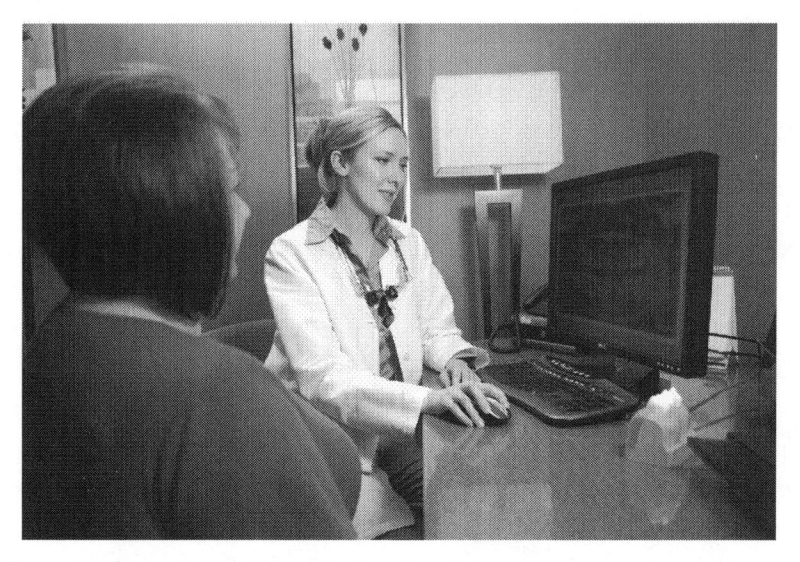

Figure 2: Create a relaxed, professional environment for your consult room.

For the Review of Findings appointment, you will need a computer and monitor or a laptop. If you are using your practice management software to display photos and radiographs, you will want to have this computer running that software.

I suggest a desk, if possible, as opposed to a working countertop, but either is OK. If you do have the resources and can get a separate monitor a little larger than the typical seventeen-inch version, that is great. Find a place in the room for models and informational material to refer to during the appointment.

Lay out the room so you and the patient are sitting next to each other, facing the monitor. In other words, avoid a situation in which you are sitting opposite each other the way you might in an operatory or when across a desk. You will find it helpful to keep a total of four chairs in the room: one for you, one for the patient, another for your assistant or front desk person, and one in the event a spouse or partner attends with your patient.

Finally, to develop your communication skills, you will want an auditory recording of your Emotional Exams, Clinical Exams, and Review of Findings appointments. This capability is a very important part of improving your approach. It is important to listen to your patient interactions on a regular basis. You will learn a tremendous amount about yourself and your patients. It is amazing how quickly you correct communication and relationship issues just by hearing yourself.

When I suggest recording appointments, some clients are concerned that the patient will object, but I have not found this to be the case. In fact, all of the dentists I work with ask their patients for permission, and in hundreds of appointments, no one has refused. At the start of each exam, simply turn on your recorder and ask the patient if she minds if you record the appointment so you do not need to take as many notes. (Please note that although you are receiving permission, you should check with your attorney for legal advice regarding recording your appointments.)

To record your appointments, I suggest an inexpensive digital recorder from your local office supply store. Whichever recording device you choose, prior to meeting with a client, make sure you know how to use it and have practiced recording and downloading. Then make sure it is placed at a distance at which the device can capture a good-quality recording.

ADRIAN WILKINS

# Preparation for an Emotional Exam, Clinical Exam, or Review of Findings

*I feel that luck is preparation meeting opportunity.*

—OPRAH WINFREY

When we learn something new, it is common for us to follow a set of instructions like the steps in a recipe. For some of us, the first few times we cook a complicated dish, we check the ingredients and the steps over and over. We do step one and then check, and then step two and so on until the dish is finished. Or for others, maybe we just get a general idea and wing it. Either way, here are a few steps to consider. Perhaps for your first appointments, before you begin, you might want to review these steps closely.

## Step 1: Intention

The mind-set you need to prepare for an operative procedure is a little different from the one you will want in the types of interactions you'll have in Emotional and Clinical Exams and Review of Findings Appointments. Here you will want to focus fully on the patients' words and thoughts rather than their teeth. Prior to the appointment, take a few minutes, and to the extent you are able to, become fully present. Perhaps perform a short four-four-eight meditation, as described in the "Going Deeper" section of "Being Present." Or if it works better for you, get in touch with your "just right moment," as discussed on page 30. And to support yourself, make sure you are not rushing into the room at the last minute. Study any patient information you might have, such as photos, radiographs, and models, ahead of time. For some people, just before entering the room, it is helpful to take a deep breath, relax, and close your eyes for a moment, remembering how much you care about your patients (this one in particular) and why you became a dentist in the first place. Then internally set your intention for this appointment. I suggest the intention be to have an organized, connected interaction with the patient, one in which she walks away feeling cared about, informed, and at choice around her dental care. Imagine the appointment going well and feeling great about the interaction.

## Step 2: Recording

As discussed earlier, start the microphone recorder just before or just as the patient is entering the room or as you are joining her. First thing, ask the patient if she would mind if you record the conversation. Let her know it will help you so you will not have to take as many notes. Patients invariably will say yes. It is important to have the recorder running before you ask so their permission is part of the recording. Thank the patient and begin.

## Step 3: Break the Ice

If it is appropriate and you are inclined, take a few minutes to break the ice with non-dental conversation. As with everything we have discussed, being real and sincere is important. Faked niceties will be experienced as just that. However, genuine interest in your patients, even if it is only about their commute, will almost always be received positively.

You might ask how they are doing today or how things have been since you last saw them. If this is the Clinical Exam or Review of Findings appointment, you've already conducted the Emotional or Clinical Exam, and you can build on other discussion topics from previous appointments. I often see dentists who see patients' family members ask how their kids are doing. Or if all else fails, the weather is a good, universal topic to get you talking.

In any case, the intent is to help the person to feel comfortable with you and continue to build rapport so she might feel at ease in choosing the best care possible for herself. It's a good time to connect with your own *appreciation* for her and to remember the intangible of truly *listening*, as you can often pick up on a patient's frame of mind right away, which will help you as you begin the appointment.

## Step 4: Frame the Appointment

Remember, most patients feel at least some anxiety about coming to see their dentist. They feel the dentist is the authority, has all of the control, and will, for the most part, dictate what happens. Even put more simply, most of us feel some sense of being unsettled when we do not know exactly what will be happening. This is one of the reasons why it's important to get patients prepared before they even arrive at the appointment. Whether you are introducing the Emotional Exam, Clinical Exam, or Review of Findings appointment, let the patient know how long the appointment will take and what to expect.

With the table set and the recipe complete, let's get into the appointments themselves. Keep in mind the principles of relationship-centered dentistry are central to all patient visits. Following are definitions and some techniques for approaching each type of exam. For each section, a diagram represents in black lettering the intangibles for success that are most supportive to focus on during the exam. These intangibles are also italicized throughout the section. It may be helpful to review each of the intangibles found in part 1 as you consider the exams.

## The Comprehensive Exam

*Diagnosis is not the end, but the beginning of practice.*

—MARTIN H. FISCHER

The Comprehensive Examination is just what the name implies. It is a thorough examination of the patient, including all of the areas you would consider treating yourself or referring to a specialist. As a reminder, the Comprehensive Exam will consist of an Emotional Exam, Clinical Exam, and photographs, all of which will support you in communicating treatment options during the follow-up Review of Findings appointment.

## The Emotional Exam

The first component of the Comprehensive Exam is the Emotional Exam. It's not found in the toolkit of exams that most offices provide, yet it is probably the most important as it relates to effective communication and success as a dentist. As such, it's important for you to be mindful of and bring in the skills of all four intangibles.

As the foundation of the Comprehensive Exam, it's the place where you learn about the person behind the teeth. Wherever possible, it should be your first appointment with the patient. This appointment can range in time between as little as

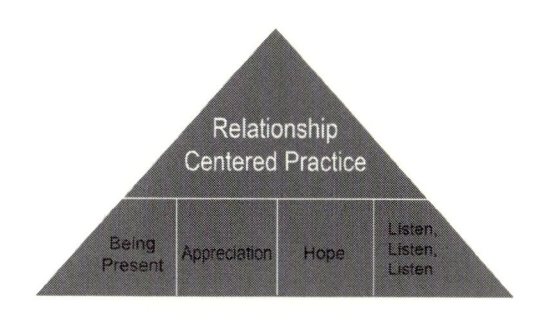

Figure 3: All four intangibles are important for an effective emotional exam.

ten or fifteen minutes to as long as an hour or more. In most cases it will be between fifteen and thirty minutes long.

This appointment is one in which the doctor speaks as little as possible and the patient as much as possible. It is an appointment that is much less about educating and much more about listening. The listening we are talking about here is for the purpose of eliciting goals, hopes, fears, attitudes, beliefs, approaches, and behaviors that impact the patient when dealing with her dental health and health in general. Although you will hopefully learn about the patient's dental condition, it is not the primary purpose of this appointment.

In addition to you learning about your patients' dental history and beliefs, there is another important benefit to this kind of appointment, that of the patients hearing themselves talk. This can be one of the most powerful things that can happen during the Emotional Exam. When the patients speak and hearing themselves speak, they often learn about themselves and reinforce their reasons for making good choices regarding their dentistry.

In fact, it can seem like magic when a patient starts to explain what has stopped her in the past from choosing the best care and then going even further to find solutions to those things that in the past had stopped them. You can imagine how much more powerful it is for a patient to identify and solve her own problem rather than being told by her dentist.

The Emotional Exam probably requires the most work to learn because it is different than what most dentists are trained to do. But once mastered, it is an invaluable tool in creating a relationship-centered dental practice.

During the Emotional Exam, interest and curiosity are focused on the emotional needs and desires of the patient. Why is she at the dentist? How does she feel about her smile? What made her choose this point in time to address her dental concerns? Does she have any dental anxiety? What does optimal oral health mean to her? How long would she like to keep her teeth? How long does she think she will keep them? The list of possible questions is endless.

The important part of the Emotional Exam is that you are *present* and interested in the human being in front of you. Your hope is to learn as much as you possibly can about the patient. One of the primary complaints of patients in dentistry and healthcare in general is that doctors and staff do not listen to them. The common experience for most patients is the doctor talking and the patient trying to get in a few words that are often either ignored or quickly dismissed. Over time, patients have come to expect doctors and staff to talk over them, and they stop trying to get their thoughts heard.

It is very powerful to watch what happens when you let patients speak. At first it is not easy; we are not accustomed to it, and the patients are not either. In the beginning, you often encounter some moments of awkward silence. But if you remain patient and ask open-ended questions that allow the patient to speak, the results are astounding. Patients will begin to tell you all of the real reasons they have put off treatment or do not come to a dentist. Very often these reasons are not the ones they share when asked short yes or no questions. The following are some more examples of open-ended questions and statements you may consider asking during the Emotional Exam.

- What brought you here today?
- Could you tell me a little bit about your past dental experiences?
- What are some of your dental goals?
- What concerns do you have about being here?
- How would you like us to support you through your care?
- When have you felt supported by dentistry?
- When has dentistry fallen short of your expectations?
- What is your understanding of a checkup?
- What is your understanding of gum disease?
- What have you done in the past to prevent gum disease?
- How did you come to decide on the treatment you have?

- ❖ You mentioned wanting whiter teeth. What do you mean by that?
- ❖ Would you expand on what having a healthy mouth means to you?
- ❖ What do you expect when you have a periodic exam and a comprehensive exam?
- ❖ What is your understanding of a regular checkup?
- ❖ How has the partnership been for you when working with a dental hygienist?
- ❖ How do you care for your mouth as a result of your partnership?
- ❖ How do you measure its effectiveness?
- ❖ What more would you like us to know about you?

Another path of questions is as follows:

- ❖ What brought you to our office today?
- ❖ What did you learn about us that helped you to decide to come to our practice?
- ❖ Could you tell me about how you have experienced dentistry in the past?
- ❖ What was treatment like for you?
- ❖ How did you come to choose the treatment you had?
- ❖ How do you feel your choices supported your goals toward achieving health?
- ❖ As you think about the goals you have for yourself, what would you like for us to pay attention to when we complete your examination today?
- ❖ What else would you like us to pay attention to that would help you feel well served?

This is just a partial list of questions, but you might find it helpful in the beginning to commit these to memory as you develop your own. With practice, asking open-ended questions will become second nature. To get a sense of how some of these questions or questions like them might be used, the following is a short example of a dentist asking open-ended questions at the beginning of an Emotional Exam:

Dentist: Good afternoon, Mary. In a little while I will bring you into the examination room and perform a Clinical Examination. Before I do that, however, I would like to spend some time with you so I can learn a little bit more about why you are here and your oral health in general.

Mary: OK.

Dentist: Mary, tell me a little bit about what brings you to the dentist today. *(Notice the request is phrased in such a way that the patient must answer with more than a yes or no.)*

Mary: I just thought I was due for a checkup, and I had some time, so I scheduled an appointment.

Dentist: Do you go to the dentist regularly?

Mary: Yes. *(Notice that this question leads to a short yes or no answer.)*

Dentist: Can you take a moment and describe your routine of going to the dentist and hygienist in the past?

Mary: Well, when I lived in Ohio, I went to the dentist every six months, but since I've been in Massachusetts, it's been three or four years since I've been. *(The question above elicits a more-detailed response from the patient.)*

Dentist: Can you tell me what the difference was between Ohio and Massachusetts?

Mary: Well, I really liked my dentist when I was in Ohio.

Dentist: Can you say more about that?

Mary: He was a really nice guy.

Dentist: (Pauses.)

Mary: He seemed really interested in me. He explained everything he was going to do, and he never hurt me. When I came to Massachusetts, I went to a new dentist, and he really wasn't very nice.

Dentist: Tell me more about the new dentist in Massachusetts.

Mary: He would just rush in and out of the room...

As you can see from the dialogue, one question leads to the next and encourages the patient to continue to expand on what she has already said. There are choices of which path the doctor will follow, but it is just that—a following of the path the patient is already on. Truly *listening* to the patient can help you follow this path. It may help you to practice the listening exercise included in the "Going Deeper" portion of the "Listening" intangible section.

During the exam, also be cognizant of *appreciating* your patients. For Mary to have made her way to your chair after having such a poor experience with her last dentist is really quite remarkable. She cared about herself enough to try again. That really speaks to our resiliency as human beings and to her courage.

Finally, though it may not be overtly spoken, be *hopeful* for her. Whatever her dental condition, she has a chance to improve it just by going through this process with you. Perhaps she will learn more about why she has avoided care in a way she hadn't understood before, and this will allow her to come back more frequently and prevent future issues. Or perhaps tangible steps will be taken toward resolving a current condition. In any case, focusing on being hopeful for her will help her to open up to you and the possibilities of regular care.

It's an important point that bears repeating: if your comprehensive exam is an hour and half long, spend at least fifteen to thirty minutes at the beginning for the Emotional Exam. During that time, your job is to listen and ask questions the way you would of a close friend you have not seen in years.

If you want to assess whether you have accomplished the intended goal of the Emotional Exam, stop and ask yourself the following questions:

- ❖ Was the doctor emotionally present and connected to himself and the patient during the exam?

- ❖ Did the patient speak at least 60 percent of the time?

- ❖ Was the conversation focused on dentistry and health goals as opposed to a large amount of unrelated small talk?

- ❖ Did the doctor come away from the exam with a clear understanding of the patient's attitudes, beliefs, goals, and objectives in terms of her health, dental, and dental-related emotional goals?

- ❖ Did the patient have moments of awareness and insight as she spoke about and explored her beliefs, attitudes, and goals?

If you can go into your Clinical Exam having answered yes to the questions above, you will be well on your way to setting the stage for a powerful doctor-patient relationship that ultimately will serve both you and the patient.

I am sometimes asked if the Emotional Exam can be performed by a team member instead of the dentist. The answer is that every team member should strive to develop the skills to conduct the Emotional Exam because these same skills and concepts should be applied throughout the patient experience.

However, I would recommend being careful about delegating this important part of your comprehensive exam to someone else. First, it can be difficult to pass the trust that is generated during the Emotional Exam to the doctor for the Clinical Exam. Second, if the team member is conducting the Emotional Exam because the doctor is not comfortable doing it, then the potential exists for that team member to leave, and when the team member leaves, a crucial skill set for the practice also leaves.

## Clinical Exam

*This diagnosis can be done in about two lines. It doesn't engage anybody.*

—DAVID FOSTER WALLACE

In general, the next step in the comprehensive exam is the Clinical Exam. The Clinical Exam is found in most typical dental practices as the New Patient Exam. The greatest difference here is that rather than the doctor examining the patient and giving the patient the doctor's findings, the doctor involves the patient in the exam.

The Clinical Exam should be a seamless continuation of the Emotional Exam. The patient should not experience a disconnect between a relationship-centered Emotional Exam to a Clinical Exam that is all about teeth, leaving the hopes and dreams of the patient behind the teeth back in the consultation room.

I'm often asked what the Clinical Exam should include. The real question is what kind of work do you perform or refer? If you perform caries control, you need to examine for caries. If you perform cosmetic dentistry, you need to examine for cosmetics. If your office offers periodontal services or endodontics or you refer out for those procedures, you need to examine for those procedures. If you treat complicated occlusion cases, you need to examine for occlusion.

What we are saying here is that every patient gets everything. The concern I hear from dentists is that this approach will take too long. If you have a lot of new patients or existing patients who need comprehensive exams, you will spend a lot of time performing exams and Review of Findings appointments. However, when you measure the time spent performing these exams compared with the productivity that generally results from this approach, it is without doubt more than worth the investment. The difference here is between being busy and being productive. Along with the Review of Findings appointment, this type of exam leads to much more comprehensive-care dentistry and therefore much more production in the dentist's schedule.

With some patients, you may choose to abbreviate portions of the exam. For example, if you perform a periodontal charting on an eighteen-year-old with excellent home care and find virtually no pocketing, you probably will not spend any additional time on a periodontal exam. If you have a patient whose occlusion looks great, you most likely will not bother with mounted models. But generally speaking, everyone gets everything.

With this approach, what I hear from doctors and patients is that the comprehensive exam acts as a way of both advertising and marketing the dentist and as a filter or a screen for attracting patients who are the right fit for the practice. When patients who do not need extensive treatment experience an Emotional Exam a thorough Clinical Exam and a Review of Findings appointment, they are often very impressed, and they communicate their perception of their dentist to their friends and family. How much do you currently pay in marketing and advertising to spread the word about the level of care you provide? What better way than getting your existing patients to do that for you?

The length of the appointment is simply a function of how long it takes you to conduct a thorough examination. Based on what I have seen working with dentists, the answer is somewhere between one hour and an hour and a half, depending on how complicated the patient is and whether the hygienist takes the full mouth series of radiographs and performs the periodontal charting. Prosthodontists and dentists who specialize in complicated cases routinely take two hours for the comprehensive exam appointment.

## Co-Discovery

The typical Clinical Exam in most dental offices consists of the dentist examining the patient and calling out his findings to his assistant. These findings are usually described in terms of procedures on tooth numbers. The type of Clinical Exam recommended here is different in that the patient is an active participant in the process.

Keeping in mind all of the information gathered during the Emotional Exam, the dentist begins to explore the patient's mouth, with the patient following along with the dentist. At the beginning of the Clinical Exam, offer the patient a mirror to hold so she can see what you see as you see it. Sometimes I am asked if you can use an intraoral camera instead of a mirror. You can; however, my preference is the mirror. When a patient is watching what is happening on a screen, it is a little less personal than looking in her own mouth. Our goal is to fully engage the patient in what is going on in *her* mouth.

As you are examining her teeth and gums, show her what you are finding. For example, you might find your explorer catch on the margin of a broken amalgam. Let the patient watch and hear what you are seeing and hearing.

Engage the patient by asking her what she sees and hears. If she asks you what it means, you can explain. For example:

Dentist: Mary can you feel and hear my explorer catching on that metal filling?

Mary: Uh-huh.

Dentist: Can you see how part of the filling is broken? Can you feel it with your tongue?

Mary: Uh-huh. Does that mean I need a new filling?

Dentist: Maybe. I am a little concerned a replacement filling may break again. I know you told me in my office that you are frustrated by always having problems and you might want to consider something more permanent.

Mary: You mean a crown?

Dentist: Possibly, but I need to study it more carefully before making a recommendation. I also heard you say cost was a concern, and I want to take that into consideration.

Mary: Yes, but I would like something that will last.

Dentist: OK, we will talk about the options during our next appointment. (Continuing with exam.) Mary, do you ever get food stuck here?

Mary: A little. Is something wrong?

Dentist: Can you see the gap between these two teeth?

Mary: Yes

The exam continues in the same way, going through the mouth tooth by tooth and looking at gums, occlusion, etc., and at the same time engaging the patient and encouraging questions. At this point, answer questions about conditions but avoid specific answers about solutions. It often becomes too complicated, and as you go through this process, you will find that you need time to come up with the best treatment options. However, sometimes it is impossible to avoid talking about solutions because the patient really insists on knowing, and in that case, avoid being too specific or definitive about recommended treatment.

You will notice in the example above that the patient is an important part of the exam. Her questions and observations help to direct the exam. Further notice how the information gathered during the Emotional Exam is integrated into the Clinical Exam.

If the patient asks about money, I recommend addressing the money questions directly, but do so in a general way and remind the patient that different options will have different costs. This approach is important because as the findings start to present themselves during the exam, money questions are natural. It also gives the patient time to start preparing mentally and emotionally for the Review of Findings appointment and avoids the element of surprise.

Finally, answer questions honestly, but where possible, explain to the patient that you really want to take some time to study the information before you can talk about it intelligently and give her the whole picture. This exam takes more patience and time than if you just recorded your findings without involving the patient. However, the benefit of making the patient part of the process is that most patients begin to own their problems, and the result is much more comprehensive-care dentistry and better patient care.

As with the Emotional Exam you will know if you have accomplished the objectives of the Clinical Exam depending on the answers to these questions:

- ❖ Was the doctor emotionally present and connected to himself and the patient during the exam?

- ❖ Was the conversation focused on dentistry and health goals as opposed to a large amount of unrelated small talk?

- ❖ Was the patient fully involved in the exam, and did she come away from the exam with a clear understanding of the conditions and problems in her mouth?

- ❖ Did the patient have moments of awareness and insight as she spoke about and explored what she saw, heard, and felt?

At the end of the appointment, schedule the Review of Findings appointment. Schedule the appointment for about a week after the Clinical Exam. This gives you enough time to study the information you gathered and gives the patient a little time to absorb the information she received in the Emotional and Clinical Exams, but it's not so long that the patient loses connection to her interest in addressing her oral health. Explain to the patient that you will study the information collected and will further discuss what you found and what can be done about it during the Review of Findings appointment.

There are a few very important points here. Stress the importance of keeping the appointment to the patient. Some patients are afraid it will mean they need a lot of work and will be pressured to do that work. Explain to them that regardless of their situations, there is no automatic expectation that they will go forward with treatment.

If there are immediate dental issues to address, explain to the patient that it is important to come because there are some immediate issues, and if she misses the appointment, these will go untreated. Tell her that your desire is to explain everything and to suggest options for treatment that are consistent with her goals and objectives.

Some dentists express a concern that the patient will not come back for the Review of Findings appointment. What I have found is that if the doctor believes in the value of the appointment and conveys that value, virtually everyone comes back for the Review of Findings appointment.

You may say something to the patient like, "Mary, when we meet next, we will discuss options for the issues we found during the exam. This may be the most important appointment we have together because this is where we together come up with a plan for you and your oral health. I would like to gear our meeting toward options for treatment that make sense for you. Everyone is different. As we talked about earlier, some people want the perfect Julia Roberts smile, and some people just want to keep their teeth. I think I generally understand what you want, but what I would ask you to do between now and when we meet is to think some more about your objectives. Specifically, what do you want in terms of dental care? And think about your budget in terms of time and money so I can focus on options that make the most sense for you."

You have now prepared her for the next appointment, and she is unlikely to cancel. She will come to the appointment relaxed because she knows you are working with her and not against her. To assist the patient between appointments, I would suggest that at some point during the Comprehensive Exam, your assistant give her a handout that tells her all of this. There is a sample in appendix 1.

When it comes to what to charge for the three exams and the photographs that comprise the comprehensive exam, it is important to understand that these appointments are not expected to be a significant source of revenue. The amount you charge is unlikely to adequately compensate you for the value you bring and the time you will spend. On the other hand, it is important to charge the patient a fee that says to the patient that this is a valuable service. With a few exceptions, I would not recommend providing this valuable service for free.

The only exception you might want to consider is if you have purchased a practice from another doctor or are part of a group practice and have inherited patients from another dentist in the practice. In those cases, you may want to consider performing some of the exams at no cost to the patient. The logic here is that it is an opportunity for you to come up to speed on a patient who already has an established relationship with the practice. Typical charges for a comprehensive exam run between $150 and $300, not including radiographs and study models.

## Photography

*One picture is worth a thousand denials.*

—RONALD REAGAN

An essential part of the comprehensive examination and Review of Findings appointment is a complete set of digital intraoral photographs. If there were only one tool I could recommend to dentists who wanted to grow their businesses, I would recommend digital photography. I will go even further to say that anyone who is not using digital photography regularly for diagnosis and communication is behind the times and risks being left behind by their competition.

Specifically, digital photography in the context of this book means intraoral photos taken with a digital camera and not an intraoral wand-type camera in hygiene. I do not object to the use of intraoral wands in hygiene for a quick review of a specific problem, but what we are talking about here is a full series of photographs with a digital camera as part of a comprehensive examination. These photos are the bridge between the Clinical Exam and the Review of Findings appointment.

Taking photographs is really the difference between explaining and actually showing the patient what you see. It allows the patient to learn to trust herself, which is far more valuable than having her trust you. In general, people remember and understand much more of what they see, hear, and collaborate on than just what is told to them. We all learn differently, so a combination of telling, showing visually, and showing again in written form will cover the spectrum of learners and native languages of patients. The more methods you can incorporate to transmit information, the better chance you will have of getting your idea across. In terms of your own education, when you are learning a new dental procedure, how much of a difference does it make to you to see it demonstrated?

If you have purchased an electronic device recently, most companies have moved away from text-only instructions. Instead, in addition or in place of manuals, company websites contain pictures and demonstrations of how to use their equipment. If you log onto YouTube, you will find thousands upon thousands of demonstrations on how to do things that have been videotaped to make learning easier.

When it comes to understanding dental needs and trusting the recommended treatment, pictures can make all the difference. This visual learning component is the reason dentists have always used wax ups, models, and drawings to explain conditions and treatments to patients.

It does take a little longer, and it can be a little more work, but the benefits of photography as an educational tool cannot be overstated. With a little practice and the implementation of a few systems, photography can become as much of a routine in your practice as taking radiographs.

If you're still a disbeliever, try this exercise. I've included a photograph in appendix 3 that I'll describe to you. Once I'm done describing it, look at the picture and tell me if you think it's what you imagined.

There's a river running left to right in the photograph. There are rocks in the foreground and trees in the background. There's a structure—perhaps a bridge?—across the river, tucked in among the trees. It has arches that go into the river. There are clouds in the sky.

How close did you get to visualizing my description? You may have gotten pieces of it, but could you visualize the interrelationship of the parts or the symmetry of the whole? If not, imagine how difficult it is for your patients when you're simply describing what's happening to individual teeth or quadrants of the mouth rather than showing them with a simple photograph.

## Taking the Photographs

While I will go over the basics, you will find a more-detailed guide describing necessary equipment and a typical shot list in appendix 2. But in brief, in addition to the camera setup, you will want wire cheek retractors, mirrors, and a protocol for taking photos.

There are quite a few good courses, videos, and books on dental photography. Depending upon how sophisticated you would like to be, you can get involved with special techniques, color balancing, and using your photos for capturing shades for the lab and printing. If you are into photography, go for it. However, we will take a more-basic approach to using photographs as a communication tool for the patient and as a diagnostic tool for you.

The first question is who should take the photographs. I have seen dentists shoot the photographs themselves with a little help from the patient holding mirrors and retractors. I have seen dentists take the photographs with their assistants and the patient holding mirrors and retractors, and I have seen assistants take the photos with some help from the patient.

The biggest issue to me is not who takes the pictures but that the pictures get taken. In almost all cases, the best-quality photos are taken by a dentist who has an interest in taking quality photos, with the help of an assistant. Some dentists really want high-quality photos, are willing to take the time to become proficient, and insist on each and every picture being of the highest quality. If that describes you, then great. You should take the photographs. My only recommendation is to not let the effort involved in taking perfect photographs get in the way of making sure it gets done. I would prefer to see average pictures taken on everyone rather than perfect pictures on just a few people.

Some dentists choose to let the assistant and patient take the photos, knowing the quality may be good but not great. They do this so photos do not require extra time on their part, and like taking radiographs, the assistant can be trained to do it without the doctor. Doing what works best for you is the key, but learn how to do it before letting someone else take over. The more comfortable you are with the process, the more likely it will become a part of your practice.

With a system and a little practice, photographs take ten minutes or less. Twelve shots can give you most of the information necessary for diagnosis and patient communication. As I said earlier, there are quite a few resources on dental photography, and if you modify the shots based on one of these other resources, it should not make much of a difference. Please see appendix 2 for the details on using photography and suggestions for appropriate shots.

## Photography Equipment

From time to time I am asked if I believe intraoral wand–type cameras are worth the expense. At this point in the evolution of dental digital photography, I do not. When intraoral cameras were first introduced, they were invaluable. At that time, digital photography was in its infancy, and the only alternative to an intraoral wand–type camera was conventional film cameras. Although a small group of dentists used them, conventional film cameras did not lend themselves to intraoral photography. Most of the cameras were heavy and bulky, and the set-up, lenses, and lighting were pretty much prototypes developed by a few technically inclined dentists. These setups generally required a fair amount of photography knowledge to make them work.

Then there was the problem of showing the photographs to the patient. For color-balancing reasons and to blow up an image, the method of choice for most dental photographs was slide film. This required having a slide-viewing system that made for an inconvenient and cumbersome way to show pictures to the patient.

Because the alternatives were not great, the wand-type intraoral camera was the best of what was available and provided a relatively fast way to show patients photos of their teeth and mouths in the environment (hygiene appointment) in which most dentists were comfortable communicating about treatment.

As dental photography technology has progressed, the tables have turned. The advantages the intraoral wand once had over conventional film photography no longer exist with newer, simpler digital cameras. Now it is generally less expensive to purchase an easy-to-use digital camera with high resolution than an intraoral wand. In addition, it is now easy to move the digital camera from operatory to operatory. As we have discussed, very little discussion of treatment should be occurring in hygiene. But even in a situation in which you want to take a quick photo in hygiene, with relative ease you can now do that with a digital camera.

A basic camera setup to take digital photographs of your patients will cost about two thousand dollars. In addition, if you do not have computers in your operatories, you will need a laptop or other computer to view the photographs with your patients. There are a number of companies specializing in digital cameras for dental photography. If you perform an Internet search for "dental cameras" or "dental photography," you will find many companies who sell complete systems.

## The Review of Findings Appointment

*I didn't realize how often I talk patients out of treatment.*

—DENTIST BEGINNING THE RELATIONSHIP-CENTERED APPROACH

Like the Emotional Exam, the Review of Findings Appointment takes place whenever possible in a consult room. This appointment is similar in some ways to what many practices call a case presentation. The major difference between the typical case presentation and a Review of Findings appointment is that this appointment is less about presenting and more about reviewing what was discovered by you and the patient during the Emotional and Clinical Exams and together confirming potential treatment options.

In the Review of Findings Appointment, you'll build off of the information learned and the trust created during the Emotional and Clinical Exams. You will review again the results of your exams and potential courses of action to resolve any issues. Expect the appointment to last about a half hour. You'll use the pictures you took during the Clinical Exam to illustrate the issues you are seeing. If you were successful in connecting with the patient and engaging her in the Emotional and Clinical Exams, then the Review of Findings almost takes care of itself.

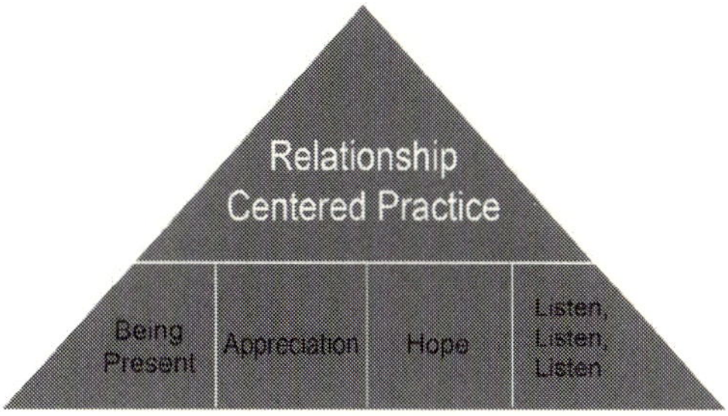

Figure 4: All four intangibles are important to practice in a Review of Findings Appointment

Throughout this process, it will be helpful to continue to remember and practice the four intangibles. At this point, the patient may be nervous because she expects to hear the bad news from both a procedure standpoint and money she will need to spend. Your *presence* is important so you don't react to the emotions she may bring in the room with her. Hopefully much of this has already been addressed prior to reaching this point in the process.

As you present your findings, *listen* to any questions she might have, and ask your own to be sure you understand where she is coming from. As you get in touch with your own *appreciation* for where she is coming from, it might help to remember a time when you were waiting for a physician to enter a room and give you the results of a test. From there, perhaps you can *appreciate* her anxiety, aloofness, or even anger, if it were to come to that. Finally, this is an important time to be *hopeful* for her so that she too can get in touch with a positive sense of improving her dental health.

The other thing we can do to help alleviate some of the patients' feelings of uncertainty is to give them an overview of what will happen during the session. Specifically, cover how long you expect the appointment to take (usually thirty minutes) and what you will be covering (e.g., aesthetics, function, structure, and biology). Repeat back to them any chief complaints or concerns they expressed to you during the comprehensive exam, and assure them you will address them. This repetition is important because patients will often tune you out if they have something to tell you that they need to get out. When you show them you heard them the last time you were together, they can relax, knowing you will address it.

Go on to explain that you will show them what you found, what it means, and the options, and together you will discuss next steps. The following is an example of that dialogue.

> Doctor: OK, Mary, when we met last I explained to you that I was going to study the information we gathered from your examination, and I have done that. What we are going to do now is take about a half hour and using the photographs and x-rays we took, take you on a tour of your mouth to review and summarize what you and I found at your last appointment. At the end of that tour, together we can talk about what the best options are for you based on your priorities.
>
> When we last met, I know you mentioned that you are bothered by the chip on your front teeth and would like to take care of that as soon as possible. I also heard you say that you have some concern about what your insurance will and won't cover. I promise we will address both of these issues.
>
> Additionally, to give you a good overview, I will be talking about aesthetics, which is what your smile looks like; function, which is the way your teeth come together—you will sometimes hear this talked about as your bite; teeth structure, which is about cavities, crowns, and fillings; and finally biology or the condition of your bones and gums. If at the end you still have questions, we can schedule more time.

And as I said before, when we are finished, we should have a plan for next steps, whether that is a treatment plan, a consult with someone else in the office, or just a plan for us to speak again. Do you have any questions about what we are going to do today?

The main point here is that the patient understands how the appointment will unfold and that you will address the concerns she expressed previously.

## Goals and Objectives

*The dentist didn't tell me about the difference between white and silver fillings until after she filled my mouth with silver. I'm so pissed. She said I could have kept more of each tooth if she had gone with white.*
—FORTY-FIVE-YEAR-OLD MAN
DISCUSSING A RECENT FILLING

Only after you have a thorough understanding of the patient's objectives can you really begin the process of describing conditions, implications, and possible solutions. Again, if you have accomplished your objectives in the Emotional and Clinical Exams, then you will know the patient's objectives clearly, and she will have a good understanding of her conditions and implications. This exam is to review anything that might not be clear from one of the prior exams and to agree on treatment options.

After framing the appointment, take a few moments and talk about the patient's objectives. Address both her needs and her wants, gauging which end of the spectrum she falls under. She may have wants-based ideas with only needs-based resources or somewhere in between, so be sure you and she fully understand her objectives.

If the patient has already told you her objectives during the prior exams, take a few minutes and repeat what you heard back to the patient until you are sure you understand. Keep in mind the patient's objectives and the chief complaint are two different things. It is important to acknowledge the patient's chief complaint, which might be a chipped tooth, as well as her overall objectives, which might be to avoid dentures.

The clearer patients and you are, the more effective the Review of Findings appointments will be. This is another critical step in the process of communicating with patients. To speak with them about their care, it is crucial for you to fully understand where they are and what they are committed to accomplish. Bear in mind that it is possible and fairly common that as patients receive and integrate new information about their situations, their objectives change.

Here is a sample of some dialogue about objectives. Notice how the dentist covers both the needs and the wants of the patient:

> Doctor: Mary, when we met last, in addition to your concerns about your chipped tooth and questions about insurance, we also discussed having me better understanding your dental priorities. I can tell you before we start that there are some decisions to be made as it relates to your oral health. It will help me quite a bit if you can give me some sense of your objectives and your budget in terms of time and money. *(It is very likely these points have already been addressed prior to this discussion.)*
>
> Patient: I am not sure I understand what you mean.

Doctor: Well, there could be a wide range of options depending on what is important to you. I would like to make sure what I suggest fits with your objectives. For example, some patients just want to stay out of pain. When a tooth breaks, they want to pull it, and eventually, they choose dentures. Other patients want a Julia Roberts smile and want to do everything they can to have perfect teeth, and there is a wide range of options between these two extremes.

I am going to explain all of those options to you, but I am going to place more attention on the ones that fit with what you tell me you would like to accomplish and your budget for doing that. The last thing I want to do is push you in a direction in which you are not interested. Does that make sense? What do you think?

Mary: I'd love to have a Julia Roberts smile, but I don't think I can afford it. I've always hated how my teeth look, but it never seemed like I could do anything about it. I don't want braces, so I've felt like I don't have any options.

Doctor: What don't you like about your teeth?

Mary: I don't like how they stick out in front and how crooked they are. My inside lip rubs against my tooth, and every once in a while, I get sores. I'd like to not have that.

By simply engaging her in a conversation, you can learn quite a bit about her priorities and even some potential needs-based work that was hidden within her wants-based explanation. Ask as many open-ended questions as necessary until you really feel you understand the patient's objectives.

## The Tour

*Those move easiest who have learn'd to dance.*

—ALEXANDER POPE

Because there are so many variables, it is difficult to describe this part of the process in a linear fashion. It is more like a dance between you and the patient that takes place throughout the relationship. However, we can identify certain aspects that are common to almost all appointments and discuss the major principles.

**Discussion Points for The Tour**
- Aesthetics
- Function
- Biology
- Structure

As you move through the Review of Findings appointment, it is important to cover aesthetics, function, biology, and structure. Present aesthetics first and then move into the areas of greatest concern. If periodontal health is a concern, still discuss aesthetics, function, and structure, but spend more time on biology.

To begin with aesthetics, show the patient her portrait photo, and follow that picture up with the lip at rest photo (see appendix 2 for full photo list). You may or may not want to point out the amount of anterior teeth she presents within the latter photo. These first photos will often elicit reactions of discomfort from patients about seeing themselves. Normalize patients' experiences by letting them know most patients feel that way.

The next photo in the presentation is the full-smile photo. Display the photograph and pause. Let her absorb seeing her smile. Since most of us do not have an opportunity to see our smiles close up this way, it would not be unusual for her to have a reaction. If she speaks, just listen.

Most healthcare professionals have a tendency to be directive in their communication. It's natural because they are the experts when it comes to their field. But as we have talked about in this book, it is much more powerful to involve the patient. Make every effort to leave space for her to talk. Listen. In this scenario, if she doesn't say anything, you may want to ask what she notices or how she feels about her smile. The more she talks, the more you understand what she knows, what she doesn't know, and where she is coming from.

If the patient indicates she has an interest in aesthetics, this is an opportunity to open that conversation. Discuss what she notices and what you notice about her smile. Avoid discussing solutions until she has indicated to you that she is interested in addressing an issue. This may be one of the most difficult changes you will have to make to utilize this approach. As discussed earlier in this book, the tendency is to say things to the patient like, "We need to do six veneers on your front teeth." Instead of talking about solutions, talk about conditions and implications. If the patient is interested in aesthetics and has said she does not like her smile, ask her what it is about her smile that she does not like. If the patient says, "My teeth are not white enough, and there is too much space between my front teeth," you might say something like, "I understand your concern." *(Notice it is her concern, not yours).* "To address the white teeth..." Given that the average person has a tooth shade of A2, show her a shade guide for what is typical, and show her where she is. If her teeth are darker, agree and suggest that if she would like to whiten her teeth, it probably will make an improvement. If her teeth are already white, tell her that, and also let her know if she would like them whiter there are things you can do.

You may address the space between her teeth by telling her you see the same thing and it also has health implications in trapping food. You might also tell her it is more noticeable because the midline is off by 3mm, drawing attention to it and indicating it should be taken into consideration with any solution. When discussing aesthetics, try to stay out of judgment and stick with pointing out the deviations from norms.

What do you do if a patient has not expressed an interest in addressing aesthetics? I suggest you still bring up aesthetics at the beginning of and throughout the Review of Findings. Simply tell the patient that you understand she is not interested in aesthetics. Let her know you will not place significant emphasis on aesthetics and you do not expect she will do anything with the aesthetics of her smile but you will give her the basic information anyway.

I suggest this method because patients who are approaching the Review of Findings from a needs-based perspective, or who are trying to avoid extensive treatment, may find when they understand what is possible that this is something they would like to address. The other reason to continue to bring it up is that many patients are somewhat embarrassed to admit that they care about aesthetics. If asked directly, they will say they do not care how their teeth look, but when given options and possibilities to improve their smile, they opt for the improvement.

Notice above that we did not suggest a solution to the patient for her aesthetic concerns. Once she has decided she wants to do something about her appearance, she will ask you how you will solve it. In the spirit of what we have discussed earlier in this book, give the patient *hope*. "We can definitely address the space between your teeth. I would suggest we apply veneers to your front six teeth. Do you know what veneers are?"

Let's explore a few more examples of how to communicate conditions, implications, and solutions. Take the example of exploring function with the patient, and suppose she has missing posterior teeth and erupted opposing teeth. You might start by asking her how she ended up with missing teeth. The "how" question is less intrusive than asking why, which tends to make a patient defensive. It is also an open-ended question that will tell you a lot about the patient. For example, you may find she has not been to the dentist because of dental anxiety.[16]

Continue the discussion by explaining that the opposing teeth are erupting and what will happen if that continues. Explain to the patient that she is compensating by chewing on other teeth, and based on the radiographs, she is losing bone because of the missing teeth. If the condition is left untreated, eventually she will lose the opposing and adjacent teeth, and it may finally become difficult or impossible to solve the problem with a nonremovable solution. Another potential implication is significant additional cost.

A word of caution here: I do not think many people have died because of missing teeth. While you should clearly point out potential implications of failing to correct a problem, do not lie, and do not exaggerate. Patients feel it and do not trust it, and it really is not necessary. Do not be afraid to say to a patient, "You can probably get away with this for quite a while." She will appreciate your honesty and will often choose to go forward with treatment either now or when she is ready in the future.

After you have explained the problem and the implications, the patient may ask you about solutions or you may need to bring up the subject. If, while you are flushing out objectives, the patient has indicated to you that cost is a serious concern, you might say to her, "The easiest, simplest, and least expensive solution is a partial denture. The major disadvantage is that it is not like having your own teeth, and you remove them at night. Some patients tell us they find it difficult to adjust to having something in their mouths, but you may find that for you it is not an issue."

---

[16] Note: You probably have noticed that the nature of these questions is similar to those found in the Emotional Exam and Clinical Exams. To a large degree, how many of these questions occur during the Review of Findings has to do with how well they were explored in the earlier exams and how much the patient absorbed.

This is opposite of the way I hear most dentists present solutions. Most start with the ideal solution and move to the less-ideal, less-expensive solution. My sense is that patients appreciate being offered the least-involved solution first. If they then say no to it, they are choosing the better option instead of hearing about the best solution, getting excited about it, and then finding out they cannot afford it. Then even the solution they do end up with is not their first choice, and there is a sense of disappointment.

In this example, let the patient know that the other option is to place dental implants. You would then explain all of the benefits and, if cost is relevant, a general idea of the cost.

This process of discussing conditions, implications, and solutions is repeated as you continue your review of patients' mouths. It is a dynamic process with give and take between the doctor and the patient. Most of the discussion should be about conditions and the implications of those conditions. In other words, there will be lots of conversation about bone loss, decay, cracks in teeth, and the consequences of having those conditions. Very little, if any, of the discussion should be about solutions. Bone grafts, fillings, and crowns should only be discussed as possible solutions after the patient understands the problem and has decided she wants to do something about it. If you think about it, it only makes sense. Until any of us decide we have a problem, need something, or want something, it really makes no sense for someone to propose a solution or suggest a purchase.

Once a patient understands her condition and the implications of the condition and has decided she would like to take action, it becomes fairly easy to come up with a solution in line with her stated objectives.

## Next Steps

Keep in mind that most people need time to make big decisions that require a significant investment. A mistake I see some dentists make is in trying to "close the deal." To begin with, there is no deal to close when you are communicating treatment from a place of integrity. Second, many patients will need time to absorb the idea of having comprehensive care. They may need to talk with a spouse or partner or to think about all of the options.

Toward the end of the appointment, remind the patient of where you started. Ask her about her objectives or remind her if she has already told you in the course of the review. Play back to her the major options—preferably two but never more than three.

Do not hand her an extensive treatment plan. Instead, handwrite the procedures she would like to do. Then open the treatment plan in the system and take a few minutes to delete the procedures she has not agreed to and give her that. Never print the treatment plan with insurance taken into consideration. Let the support staff give her those specifics. This has the advantage that when the insurance is factored in, the price goes down a little. Because it is an improvement over her expectations, this price decrease will of course be a plus to the patient.

Let the patient know that you understand this is a big decision and that unless a portion of the treatment has a specific urgency, it is better for her to take her time to decide. What I would suggest, though, is that you get a sense from her about where she is and agree on the next step. You might address this with her simply as, "How do you feel about what we've discussed today? And do you have any sense of the next step you'd like to take in your process?" Again, this is not to close the deal but to get a sense of her thought process. As you get into the discussion with her, you could reflect back to her what you think she's telling you about the next step in her process. Some possible next steps include:

❖ Schedule for treatment.

❖ Print a treatment plan, and have the treatment coordinator review it in detail.

- ❖ Arrange financing.

- ❖ Schedule for a consult with a specialist.

- ❖ Set up a second consult to give the patient time to think about what she would like to do.

- ❖ Set her up to speak with an administrative person about finances. Make sure the administrative person completes with a next step of his own.

- ❖ Schedule one small procedure to get a feel for working with you. This can be helpful for a phobic patient or someone who needs some restorative work regardless of other choices. This often is an easy thing for the patient to say yes to, and when she comes back, she has had time to absorb the Review of Findings appointment. Do not use this approach as a way to get the patient back in without doing a separate Review of Findings. You need to become comfortable with the value of the Review of Findings appointment.

- ❖ Have her agree to receive a call from your front desk or administrative person to follow up. Reassure the patient that if she cannot or does not want to go forward with treatment that is OK, but you want to stay in touch with her to plan next steps.

- ❖ Speak with her spouse or set up an appointment with a spouse to review.

Before she departs, repeat the next step to be taken, such as, "As we discussed, you'll be hearing from my office within the next week to follow up." This will ensure you're both on the same page. At this point, acknowledge her for her willingness to follow the process through fully, as it is certainly the best way you know to keep a healthy smile.

## Periodic and Emergency Exams

In this model, Hygiene and Emergency exams support the goal of delivering comprehensive dental care. The Hygiene and Emergency exams allow you and your staff time to bond with the patient and gain trust, and in most cases, they are steps toward a Comprehensive Exam.

## Periodic Exam/Hygiene Check

In many offices, periodic exams or hygiene checks are the primary appointments (other than the new patient exam) to examine and present treatment. In a relationship-centered approach, this exam should be about communicating the need for a big-picture exam and a view of the patient's situation. For a number of reasons, this is not the best time to examine a patient for comprehensive needs, the obvious reason being that there is not enough time to do it thoroughly.

If you are fortunate and able to gain enough information to understand what is going on, it does not allow sufficient time to communicate those needs in detail. Even if you are able to understand and communicate enough information to the patient so she understands the situation and the potential solutions, there is still a problem. Very few patients have the psychological and emotional makeup to come to a decision on the spot. Since we are suggesting that a periodic examination is not the right time to examine for or present comprehensive treatment, what should happen instead?

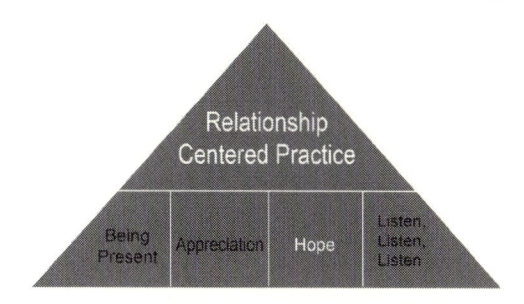

Figure 5 Three of the four intangibles are important to emphasize during a Periodic Exam/Hygiene Check

In most offices I work with, I am told that the periodic exam lasts between five and ten minutes out of a one-hour hygiene appointment. What I see in practice is that the periodic exam is often less than five minutes. Within such a short amount of time, the periodic exam should accomplish the following.

- ❖ First, establish, solidify, and build on your rapport and relationship with the patient. This is an important time to remind yourself what you like about this patient and express that to her. Remember that *appreciation* is one of the intangible keys to connecting with your patients. *Listen* carefully to the patient, and clarify where she is mentally. How prepared is she to bring her mouth back to optimal health? This does not mean convincing the patient to do something but rather listening, understanding, and relating to the patient where she is today.

- ❖ Second, do an oral cancer screening so your patients receive this valuable service at least every six months.

- ❖ Next, review any major concerns of the patient, review new findings by the hygienist, and check where the patient is in terms of existing treatment plans.

- ❖ Finally, if the patient has not had a new patient exam or has not had a comprehensive exam in the last four to five years (usually coinciding with a full-mouth series of radiographs), the time is spent explaining to the patient why it is in her best interests to come in for a comprehensive exam.

- ❖ You may say something to the patient like, "Mary, it has been a few years since we performed a comprehensive exam on you. There seem to be a few things developing, and it would be smart right now to have a thorough examination and make a plan for the next few years." Or it might be more urgent. "Mary, I am seeing a number of things going on that concern me, and I don't feel we can adequately address them in this short examination. My suggestion is that you come back and we spend the time and give you a thorough examination."

This exam is really just about establishing and building upon your relationship with the patient and communicating a view of her situation and the need for a big-picture exam. When a patient understands the reason and value of a comprehensive examination, it is rare that she will reject it.

## Emergency Exam

*There is nothing so strong or safe in an emergency of life as the simple truth.*

—CHARLES DICKENS

Emergency exams are similar to the hygiene check in that besides dealing with the immediate issue, this exam can be utilized to explain to the patient why it is in her best interest to come back for a comprehensive examination. This is not the time to go into detail regarding everything going on in the patient's mouth. This is a good time to tell her that there are some issues that will require her to make some decisions and to suggest she come back for the comprehensive exam.

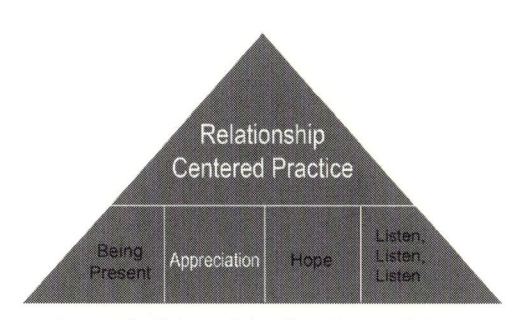

**Figure 6 Three of the four intangibles are important to emphasize in an Emergency Exam.**

Emergency patients can present a specific problem in that many of them are in for an emergency because they have not been keeping up with care and to some extent, have been avoiding their problems. If this is the case, it often helps to assure patients that coming in for a comprehensive exam does not mean they are immediately going to need a lot of work or that you will push them into treatment for which they are not ready. They may need to be educated that getting the information and developing a plan is something that really is in their best interest. In addition, some patients think they are beyond hope. One way of inspiring hope in this type of patient is to focus on the fourteen healthy teeth rather than the fourteen unhealthy teeth. Let them know that no matter what the problem, in most cases, a plan can be developed that over time will address their needs, and the most important step to future health is to come in for the comprehensive examination.

From a relationship-centered/comprehensive-care standpoint, here are a few things to consider for emergency exams.

- ❖ This appointment is about *being present* with patients, building relationships, and helping them to find *hope*.

- ❖ You can support the patient in building *hope* by being straightforward, helping to lessen her fear by letting her know that her problem can be solved, and painting a vision of what's possible.

- ❖ This appointment is a time to *listen* and ask questions that help you to understand the patient and to let her know you really care about her. You might ask her how the problem arose and then just listen. Very often a patient will tell you a story that provides you with invaluable information that explains why she is where she is. Once you have that knowledge, it is much easier to support her in getting the right care.

## Establishing Value for the Comprehensive Exam

During both the periodic and emergency exams, one of your main objectives is to create value and prepare the patient for what to expect in the comprehensive exam. Included in appendix 1 of this book is a sample handout to give your patients when scheduling them for it. This scheduling should occur during their periodic or emergency exam. The purpose of the handout is to reinforce the difference between typical exams they've experienced and a comprehensive one. It also lets them know the appointment length and what to expect, and it reassures the patient that having the exam is not an automatic indication she will need or be pressed to accept comprehensive treatment. The handout also alerts the patient to the fact that she will have an additional Review of Findings appointment after the comprehensive exam.

In chapter 5, we discussed how to put it all together. We discussed each exam and the Review of Findings appointment and how they support a relationship-centered approach to dentistry. Earlier we talked about the Platinum Rule of treating others as they would like to be treated. In chapter 6, we'll look at how to quickly determine how a patient would like to be treated based on how she presents herself.

## Summary of Key Points

- *Relationship-Centered Dentistry.* Practicing this way requires a different structure than the traditional dental practice.

- *Set the Table.* Prior to meeting with your patients, prepare yourself and your space to support you and them. When you begin the appointment, break the ice so they feel comfortable with you, and frame the appointment so both of you are on the same page.

- *Comprehensive Exam.* The Comprehensive Exam consists of the Emotional Exam, the Clinical Exam, Photographs, and a Review of Findings Appointment. They are foundational pieces of Relationship Centered Dentistry.

- *Hygiene and Emergency Exams.* In addition to addressing urgent needs, use these appointments to build rapport and develop value for a Comprehensive Exam.

- *Photography.* Photography is an invaluable tool for creating awareness and trust and may be one of the most-important capabilities you can add to your practice.

**CHAPTER 6**

# Additional Tools

## Meeting Patients Where They Are

*You want to work with people who you like and have an easy rapport with.*

—MIKE WHITE

Most of what has been discussed in this book falls under the umbrella of relationship building. A solid doctor/patient relationship will turn any practice into a successful business. Imagine how it would feel if your patients truly looked forward to seeing you. What if they felt seen and heard by you and empowered in your office? As a result, these patients would happily come to your office to be in your presence. It is possible to be so genuinely with a patient that she makes the first move, coming to you with what dental care she would next like to engage in based on the information you have shared about her oral health.

So what's the magic trick? There isn't one, really. If you are present and connected and are supporting your patient with the four intangibles (Being Present, Hope, Appreciation, and Listen, Listen, Listen) as I've referred to throughout this book, the rest will happen naturally; however, there are tools that can make it easier for you to make that connection with your patients. These tools allow you to match your language and communication style to each client while maintaining your personal integrity—projecting the essence of who you are in a way the patient can easily relate to.

Learning about how we are different from each other will open up the possibility for you to be a better communicator. Seeing the people who are in front of you, rather than perceiving them as an extension or mirror of yourself, means you are meeting them where they are. You are being with them and accepting them. If you've ever had a conversation with someone in which you left feeling he or she truly got you, that's what I mean.

This explicit acceptance of your patients will allow them to leave your office feeling better about themselves than when they came in, and most of us would like a taste of that.

## CAPS Model

To support you in communicating with your patients, I recommend using a personality matrix based on the CAPS model, developed by David W. Merrill, PhD, and Roger H. Reid, MA.[17] The model below is loosely based on their system.

This system utilizes a test to determine one of four major personality types. The only drawback to this system is that the style distinctions are not granular, but an advantage to this system is that a self-test, though recommended

---

17  Merrill, D. W., and Reid, R. H. *Personal Styles and Effective Performance*

for accuracy, is not necessary. By the time you have completed a client's first comprehensive exam, you will be able to make an assessment about two traits.

- *Is the patient Dominant* (Extroverted, Assertive, Direct, Talkative) *or Easy Going* (Introverted, Passive, Subtle, Quiet)?

- *And does the patient present herself as Formal* (Proper, Reserved, Organized, dresses and speaks more formally) *or does she seem Informal* (Relaxed, Laid back, Spontaneous, dresses and speaks informally)?

You can see in the following chart how determining whether someone is dominant, easygoing, formal, or informal determines which of the four personality types the patient falls under.

Dominant/Formal = Controller
Easygoing/Formal = Analyzer
Dominant/Informal = Promoter
Easygoing/Informal = Supporter

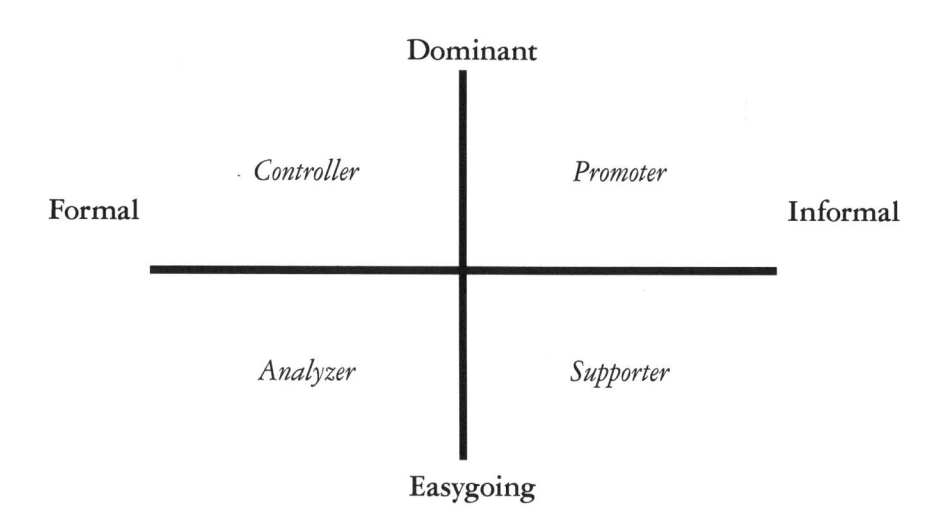

```
                    Dominant
                       │
         Controller    │    Promoter
Formal                 │                Informal
───────────────────────┼───────────────────────
         Analyzer      │    Supporter
                       │
                    Easygoing
```

The following section describes each of the traits of these personality types and how, in general, to relate to them.

## Dominant, Formal—Controller

- ❖ Task accomplisher
- ❖ Bottom-line results
- ❖ Self-motivated
- ❖ Forward looking
- ❖ Fast decision-maker
- ❖ Initiates activities
- ❖ Disciplined
- ❖ Likes to control others
- ❖ Lots of eye contact

Controllers stereotypically are your type-A, driven patients. They are often executives or in other positions of power. They tend to be direct and to the point and are not very interested in personal relationships. Typically they are looking for competence, not friendship, and they make decisions quickly and easily. In addition to the clues described above, they tend to focus on "what" questions, like, "What is the point of that?"

*Relating to Controllers*

- ❖ Let them be in charge
- ❖ Be businesslike
- ❖ Do not expect friendship
- ❖ Staff and doctor need to be competent and efficient
- ❖ Very little small talk
- ❖ Once *they* make a decision, they can act quickly

When relating to a controller in a dental practice, it is important to be to the point in your communication. The approach in this book works well with controllers in that you give them the information, and they will make a decision. They are generally more comfortable when the solution is their idea and do not respond well to being told what to do.

*Examples of Controllers*: Donald Trump, General Patton, driven CEOs

## Easygoing, Formal—Analyzer

- ❖ Objective
- ❖ Conscientious
- ❖ Defines, clarifies
- ❖ Concerned with accuracy
- ❖ Gathers needed data/information
- ❖ Tests data
- ❖ Maintains standards
- ❖ Very little visible emotion
- ❖ Little physical contact
- ❖ Little eye contact

Analyzers are your stereotypical engineers, accountants, and technicians of one type or another. Analyzers want to understand the details. They are methodical and logical and tend not to be very emotional. Like controllers, they respect competence. In addition to the clues described above, they tend to focus on "why" questions, like, "Why are you suggesting the root canal before the crown?"

*Relating to Analyzers*

- ❖ Be logical
- ❖ Give them lots of information

- ❖ Demonstrate technical competence
- ❖ Talk facts, not opinions
- ❖ Do not push them for quick decisions
- ❖ Appeal to the rational instead of emotional side of them
- ❖ Don't make them wrong

When it comes to relating to analyzers, it is best to keep giving them information. Unlike promoters, who are likely to throw out the flyer on periodontal health, analyzers will study it and then go to the Internet for more. Analyzers will often appear to be avoiding making a decision by asking for more and more information. Be patient. Do not push an analyzer to make a decision.

*Examples of Analyzers:* Stephen Hawking, Mr. Spock, scientist types

## Dominant, Informal—Promoter

- ❖ High energy
- ❖ Enjoyable to be around
- ❖ Creative imagination
- ❖ Initiates relationships
- ❖ Motivating
- ❖ Competitive spirit
- ❖ Goal oriented
- ❖ Emotional
- ❖ High animation

Promoters are fun-loving people who are the life of the party. They usually come bouncing through the front door and immediately engage in conversation with the staff and doctor. They tend to relate emotionally and are big-picture people. Unlike controllers, they care about your competence, but they also want to know that you care about them. In addition to the clues described above, they tend to focus on "how" questions, like, "How will you do that?"

*Relating to Promoters*

- ❖ Be enthusiastic
- ❖ Relate emotionally
- ❖ Paint the vision
- ❖ Acknowledge them for making good decisions
- ❖ Create a strong support system for them to follow through.

When relating to a promoter, show enthusiasm. Have fun. Paint the vision as well as explain the facts. This can be a stretch for some dentists, who can be somewhat analytical. But the more expressive you are and the more you relate on an emotional level, the more the patient will feel seen and cared about.

*Examples of Promoters:* Tony Robbins, Mary Lou Retton, cheerleader types

## Easygoing, Informal—Supporter

- ❖ Dedicated and committed
- ❖ Loyal team member
- ❖ Good listener
- ❖ Patient
- ❖ Good at reconciling factions
- ❖ Cause-oriented
- ❖ Dependable
- ❖ Relationships mean a lot
- ❖ Shows when they are pleased, not when unhappy
- ❖ Lots of physical contact

Supporters are very warm, loving people. They can be a little on the quiet side, but they are very caring and appreciate when people care about them. They tend to agree with the statement, "People don't care how much you know until they know how much you care." They are genuinely interested in you and your family. Once they trust you, they are very loyal. They may have difficulty making a decision. In addition to the clues described above, they tend to focus on "who" questions, like, "Who will be doing the treatment?"

*Relating to Supporters*

- ❖ Relate on an emotional level
- ❖ Build a relationship
- ❖ Encourage their thoughts
- ❖ Sometimes you will need to be fairly direct in guiding them.
- ❖ Don't be surprised if they go home and their spouse influences them
- ❖ It may be helpful to meet with spouse, parent, etc.

Supporters can be a little tricky to work with. Since they tend to base their decisions on whether they trust and like you, in some ways they are easy to work with. Just genuinely care about them, and they will listen. The problem comes in that since they trust you, they are often the ones who will just tell you to do what you think is best. I highly recommend making a strong effort to make sure they understand and are going forward with treatment from a place of commitment, not compliance. You may also find it helpful to have their spouse or significant other at the Review of Findings appointment because they will often have a lot to do with treatment decisions.

*Examples of Supporters:* Mother Theresa, nurses, motherly/grandmotherly types

## How to Use Personality Information

The intention of this model is not to pigeonhole any of your patients into a static category. Rather, this simplified assessment tool attunes your relational style to match your patients. This formula will support your ability to speak their language and match their energy while staying true to who you are and remaining in integrity. This is a "fake it 'til you make it" mechanism that will allow you to meet your patients where they are as you learn to be with them.

I suggest that you integrate this tool into your practice by meeting with your staff and teaching everyone in your office how to identify these personality types. One way to do this is to practice on each other and ask the people in your office to do this with everyone they meet for a week. It does not take long to get good at it.

In many offices, the person taking the intake call or the person at the front desk will use his initial observations to determine what language your patient speaks. I have some offices that then mark the chart C, A, P, or S to indicate the personality type. This is just a best guess that is then verified by the rest of the team and the doctor. Keep in mind this system is not as precise as something like the Myers-Briggs system, and people will often fall between two personality types, so for example, someone may be a controller/promoter. You will notice, however, that in most cases, people will not be a combination of opposite corners on the chart above.

Once you know how to speak the patients' language, and once you have become adept at speaking to each of these personality types, you will likely find it to be a powerful tool to help you relate to the people coming through your door. Offices frequently tell me this is one of the most valuable things they use.

Like everything offered in this book, these guidelines provide useful tools. What is also true, though, is that as much as the technique and approach will make a dramatic improvement, there is no substitute for the intangibles I described earlier. And as much as I would like to be able to give you a guaranteed cookbook, this process will be most successful if you are able to connect with yourself and your patient by being present, giving evidence of your appreciation, offering hope, and listening.

It's like the difference between a dentist with good hands and a good feel compared to a dentist who does not have that touch. Each dentist uses the same equipment, supplies, and technique, but one can just do it better than others.

So, how do you make the most of every conversation? Where you are coming from? This may be the most important question one can ask oneself in human relations. This is the question that can cause us to look at ourselves to the extent we are able in an honest way. This question does not deal specifically with what words to use, what questions to ask, or techniques in communication. It deals instead with identifying our personal agendas when relating to others.

It is the question that, when answered, reveals our intention. Am I coming from a place of understanding when I speak to a patient, or am I coming from a place of judgment? One can ask the same question from a place of judgment instead of understanding, and the exact same question can have very different meanings. For example, take the simple question, "How did you lose those teeth?"

Coming from a place of understanding, you can see the dentist, hygienist, or assistant asking the question and being genuinely concerned about the patient. These people probably have compassion and curiosity that invites the patient to share safely how she got to this place in her life.

On the other hand, if they are coming from a place of judgment, it will sound very different to the patient. The quality of disconnection and lack of understanding can cause the patient to hear the question as a statement that she is bad or wrong for having allowed this to happen.

Depending on your agenda, it is also possible for the patient to hear the question as having more to do with your needs than hers. Perhaps the message she hears behind the question is, "Here is an opportunity for me to sell implants," or, "Is this a way to pay the rent this month?" Whatever your intention is in your communication, it cannot be hidden fully. The patient will take in the energy of the message more than the words themselves.

All of what I have said here partially ignores that patients also play an important part in terms of how they hear what you say to them. We do not have control over the filter other people hear through (assuming we do would be caretaking). It is possible that you could be coming from a very compassionate and understanding place and the patient will hear it through the filter of judgment.

For the most part, people will hear and feel where you are coming from. You know this is true based on your own experience. You know when a person is smiling in that patronizing way and telling you he would be happy to help you, yet you know underneath that is the furthest thing from his mind. And you know how it feels when the person is genuine in his communication.

As I already mentioned, a majority of communication is nonverbal. This nonverbal communication is generated by where we are coming from. It is relatively easy to fake words, but it is almost impossible to fake our energy or our personal agenda. Be conscious of your intentions, be compassionate with yourself and your patients, and see where it takes you.

## Summary of Key Points

- *Everyone Is Different.* Each of us is different and speaks a different language. Knowing each other's language goes a long way to creating a relationship.

- *The Platinum Rule.* Treat others as they would like to be treated, not as you would like to be treated.

# CONCLUSION

I am completely convinced that effective communication through a commitment to relationship-centered dentistry is the cornerstone of a successful and fulfilling comprehensive-care dental practice. The temptation to look for the next marketing gimmick or to add another service to your repertoire is great; the hope is that there is an easy way to bring in the right type of patient. Marketing and advertising are essential to a healthy practice, but without effective communication, they alone do not guarantee these patients will understand and choose comprehensive care.

The thought of committing yourself to developing your communication skills can seem daunting, and for some people, it can feel unattainable. Many of us believe you need to be born with this innate talent and it is out of reach for the rest of us. So far I have not met anyone who cannot make a dramatic improvement in his or her ability to communicate effectively. It requires the knowledge that I believe this book provides. It also requires commitment and practice, of which all of us are capable.

The benefits of this approach are nothing less than amazing. I have seen dentists take practices in which they struggled to survive and turn them into highly successful businesses. I have watched dentists move from single-tooth dentistry to quadrant and full-mouth dentistry almost exclusively through their commitment to effective communication.

More important than the financial rewards has been watching one dentist after another tell me they are finally enjoying their patients again. The experience of authentic, connected communication in and of itself is truly the reward of this process.

I hope you have learned enough in this book to convince you to give this process a try. In any case, I wish you many years of enjoyment and success in the world of dentistry.

**APPENDIX 1**

# Hygiene Check, Periodic Exam, and Emergency Exam Handout

**ADRIAN WILKINS**

# Comprehensive Examinations

**How a comprehensive examination benefits you.**
One of the best ways to avoid extensive dental treatment and the costs associated with extensive treatment is by having a comprehensive plan or road map for improving and maintaining your oral health. When you have a comprehensive examination, your dentist, working together with you, can develop a plan that meets your dental objectives, factoring in common considerations such as time and money. This way you have control of your oral health and can avoid unexpected and costly surprises.

**Who should get a comprehensive exam and how often?**
From the patient with minimal dental needs to the person with extensive needs, everyone benefits from a comprehensive examination and a review of findings. Patients with minimal needs should expect to have a comprehensive examination every four to five years. Patients with more-complicated situations should plan on at least every three years. In all situations, the comprehensive examination is that ounce of prevention that avoids a pound of cure.

**How does a comprehensive examination differ from a checkup (periodic) examination?**
A periodic examination is a relatively short examination during which your dentist performs a brief examination of your gums and teeth. Your doctor will perform an oral cancer screening, and your hygienist will take the appropriate x-rays. However, the periodic examination is not the examination in which your dentist determines your overall needs. Instead, he or she uses your last comprehensive examination as a starting point and uses the periodic exam to make sure you are on the right track.

The comprehensive examination is more extensive and is the foundation for a big-picture plan for your oral health. This is the time we generally recommend getting a full-mouth series of x-rays, photographs, periodontal charting, study models if necessary, and a detailed examination by your dentist. This exam is followed by a review of findings appointment (which is included in the cost of the exam). Between the comprehensive exam and the review of findings appointment your dentist will study your x-rays, photographs, and other diagnostic information. When you meet, your doctor will show you what he or she has found, and together a plan will be formulated that best suits your situation. A comprehensive examination may be the most important thing you as a patient can do to maintain your oral health.

## Review of Findings Appointment: About Your Next Visit

Your next visit will last approximately half an hour. During that visit, you and your doctor will sit and discuss what he or she found during your comprehensive examination. Unless your doctor has told you differently, you are unlikely to have any dental treatment during that visit.

Between now and your next visit, the doctor will review the x-rays, photographs, and other diagnostic information collected during your examination. The doctor will then come up with a number of potential treatment options to discuss with you when you meet. The fee for this is included in the comprehensive examination, and there is no additional charge for this visit.

**Why Do We Schedule a Separate Appointment?**

Traditionally dentists have examined the patient and made recommendations in the same appointment. This is not ideal because the doctor does not have the time to study all of the possible options, and there is simply not enough time to explain to the patient what is happening in his or her mouth.

We schedule a separate appointment to give the doctor time to review all of the information collected during the examination and develop options that fit with your objectives. And most importantly, it gives the doctor time to sit with you and show rather than tell you about what he or she has found. The fact that we are scheduling a second appointment does not necessarily mean you need extensive work. Almost all of our patients who receive a comprehensive examination are invited back for a review of findings appointment.

It is very important to keep this appointment because if you miss it and have any acute problems requiring attention, these problems will go untreated. If you need to cancel this appointment, it is important that you reschedule.

## What We Need from You

In some dental offices, patients leave the dentist feeling pressured about treatment. Often this is because the dentist is suggesting optimal treatment, and that is not what the patient wants or can afford. The result is the dentist encouraging the patient to do something that is not right for him or her.

At [insert name of your dentistry here], we are committed to giving our patients the best dentistry possible that fits within our patients' objectives. To do that, between now and your next visit, we ask you to think about your goals for your oral health and your budget in terms of time and money to accomplish those goals. For example, some patients simply want (or can only afford) to stay out of pain until their teeth are removed and replaced with dentures. Others would like the perfect cosmetic smile.

At our office, we have an obligation to provide quality dental care and diagnosis. However, we will do everything we can to recommend treatment that makes sense in terms of your goals and your budget. Between now and your appointment, think about what is right for you.

## Dental Insurance

Dental Insurance is often a part of treatment decisions, and it can be very confusing. If you are interested in learning more about dental insurance, feel free to ask any of our business staff.

**APPENDIX 2**

# Photography Guide

This basic set of photos is typically sufficient to create a baseline record for the patient, for use by the dentist to study the case, and as a presentation tool. As I have already mentioned, taking these exact photos is not critical.

Once you have your photographs, they will be on a memory card in the camera. I suggest getting a few memory cards since they are very inexpensive. You can download your pictures directly from your camera by plugging the camera into your computer. Instead, I would recommend getting an inexpensive card reader and attaching it to the computer to which you are downloading the pictures.

By doing it this way, you can take the card out of the camera and the card will contain the photos for that specific patient. You will then either download the photos onto your computer in a third-party program (Picasa from Google is a free download that is easy to use and works well) for viewing or editing, or you will download the photos into your practice-management software. The major practice-management programs all have tools for downloading and editing patient photographs. One note of caution: Make sure when you are shooting the photographs that your camera is set for a relatively small file size. Unless you are using the photographs for lecturing, you do not need anything big, and if you are not careful, you will eat up large amounts of space on your computer system.

Once you have downloaded the photographs to your computer, either you or your assistant will want to flip the pictures that were shot using a mirror because these pictures will be backward. In addition, you may want to crop or blow up areas for better viewing. And finally, you want to put them in order for your Review of Findings appointment. For example the last shot you took was the portrait shot, but it will probably be first for your presentation.

The important thing here is to come up with an easy system for downloading, cropping, and preparing photos for your Review of Findings appointment. If at all possible, I highly recommend training your assistant or another technically savvy person in the office to take this task off your shoulders. The easier it is to do, the more likely you are to do it. It generally takes people a while to come up with a system, but once they do, it becomes a routine process.

//THE WAY OF THE SUPERIOR DENTIST

# Photography Guide

<u>Tools you will need:</u>
Camera
Mirrors
Retractors
Warm Water

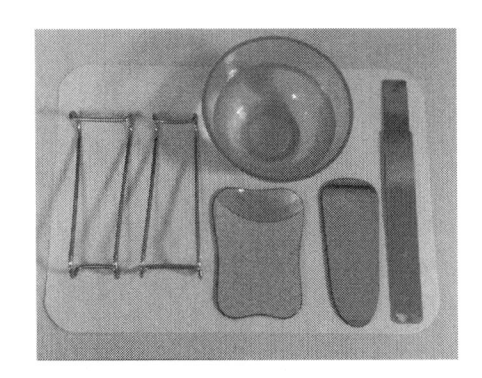

<u>Introduction:</u>
The objective of these instructions for taking a Comprehensive Series of Photographs is to create a consistent, comprehensive, and quick way to capture images for the purpose of patient co-diagnosis and communication. A thoughtful dialogue and presentation can reduce patient resistance and increase the efficiency and the quality of the images taken. Each image has a diagnostic objective. You may want to add or subtract images to suit your own objective. In this guide we take 14 images; they can be completed by one person in approximately 5 minutes. You will want to consult your instruction manual for ISO, shutter, f-stop, and flash settings. In the photos below, you will see a picture on the left showing how the photo is taken and the result you are trying to achieve on the right. Note: During the intake process and prior to the exam, a consent form for diagnostic radiographs and photographs is presented.

<u>Full Smile Straight:</u>
The first thing to say to the patient is, "The first 3 photographs are going to be of your smile, so I want you to give me a big smile showing your teeth." Some patients will resist and say, "I don't smile that way or at all." Follow with, "I understand, but what I am really trying to see is how much tooth or gum you show if you were to really smile big." The camera is first held parallel and level to the patient's eyes and centered to the midline, framing

the lips corner to corner, then drop down being sure to stay parallel to the plane of occlusion. At this point, say, "You may want to close your eyes now because a flash is coming."

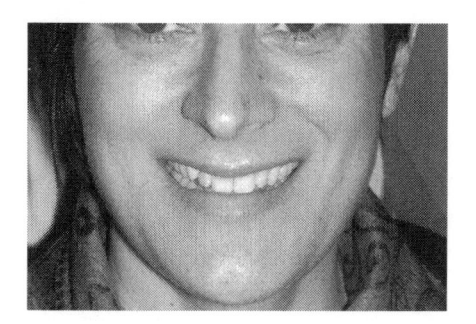

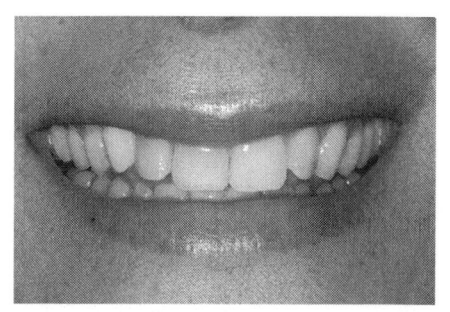

## Full Smile Right:
Move slightly to the patient's right side and focus on the upper lateral incisor and say, "Here comes the next smile photo."

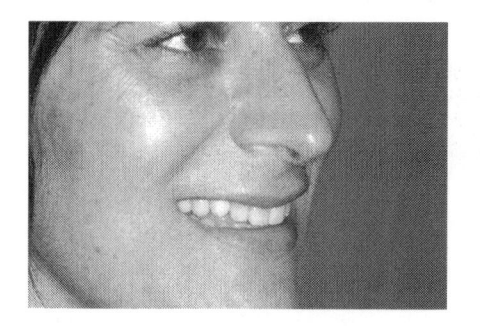

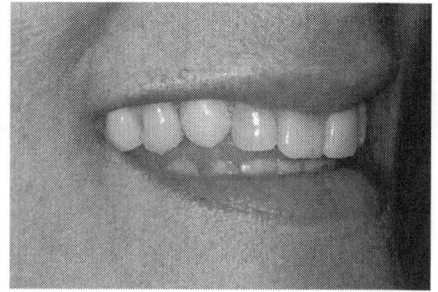

## THE WAY OF THE SUPERIOR DENTIST

### Full Smile Left:
Now move to the left side of the chair and have the patient continue smiling and say, "Last smile photo."

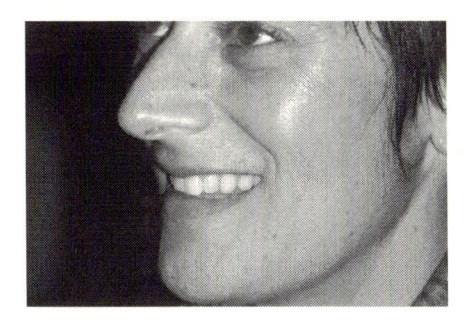

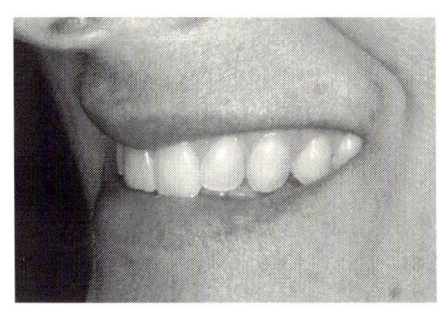

### Lip at Rest:
"Now I want you to completely relax your face." At this point, gently touch the patient's face with your fingers, and when you feel the patient is completely relaxed, say "Now just slightly drop your chin open."

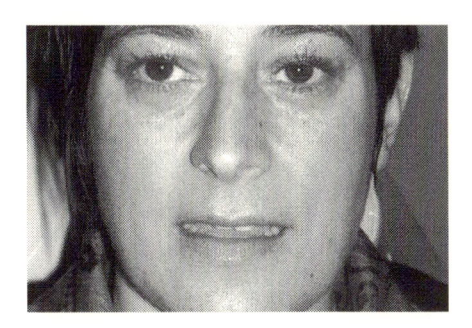

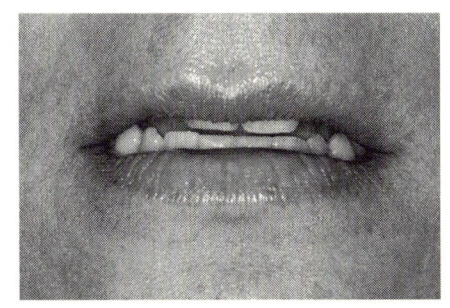

### Retracted Closed:
The next 3 photographs in this series are centered and retracted views. Depending upon the flexibility of the lips, you may want to experiment briefly with the small and large ends of the retractors. You want to be able to

see as much cervical gingiva as possible. On some occasions, you may want to switch to clear plastic retractors which may retract much more fully, but they are much more difficult to place. Once you have decided which end to use, hold the retractors firmly in front of the patient and ask that the patient to hold them exactly the same way. Place the holders in the lips and transfer the grip to the patient. Patients will often hold the retractors more symmetrically than an assistant holding them from the side. Again, be certain to be level with the plane of the eyes and the plane of occlusion, and tell the patient, "Close down on all of your back teeth."

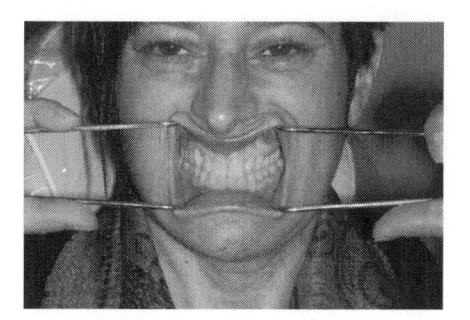

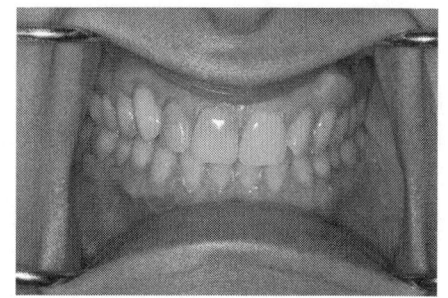

### Retracted Open:
Staying in the same position, tell the patient, "Open just a little until I tell you to stop." When you see the entire edge of the lower arch, take your photo.

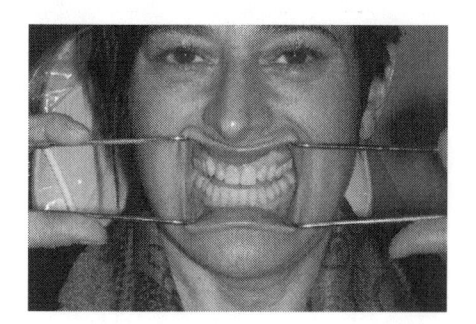

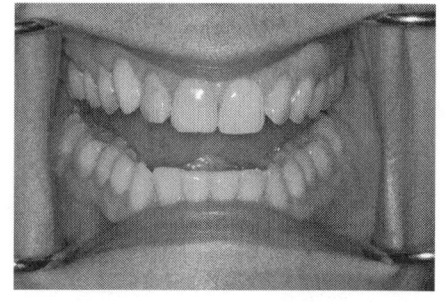

## Anterior Edge to Edge:
Now tell the patient, "Slide your front teeth edge to edge."

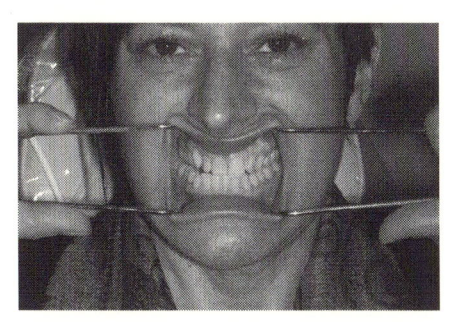

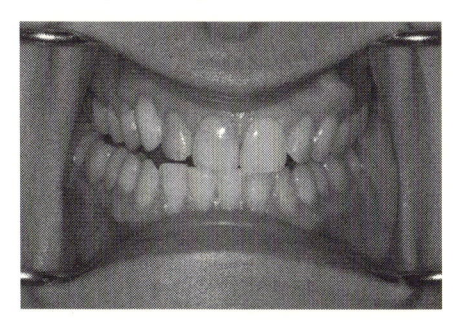

At this point, ask the patient to remove the retractors and hold onto them for a moment while you prepare the mirrors for the next shots.

## Upper Arch Occlusal:
Warm the mirror in the water bath and completely dry the mirror. Now tell the patient to place the small end of the retractors in his or her mouth. The small end works better on occlusal views. Instruct the patient, "Tip your head way back and open as widely as you can." Place the back end of the mirror on the distal sides of most posterior teeth and hold in the center. If the lips cover any part of the occlusal arch, get the patient to pull upward until the teeth are exposed.

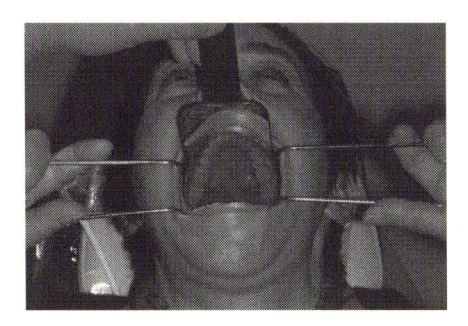

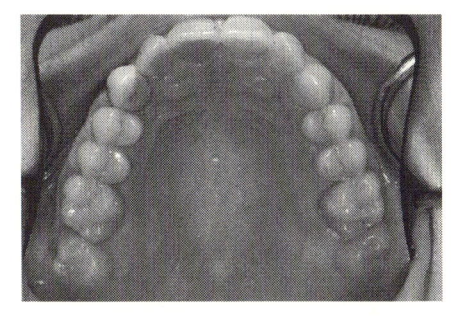

Note: After downloading this photo, in order to get the correct orientation, you must rotate 180 degrees and mirror the image using your photo imaging software.

## Lower Arch Occlusal:
Now do the same on the lower arch, and ask the patient to tip the head down and open wide.

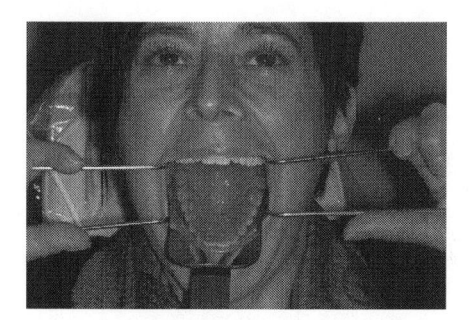

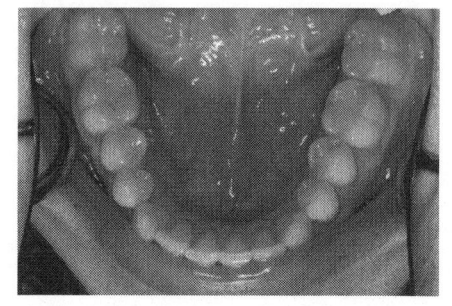

Note: After downloading this photo, in order to get the correct orientation, you must rotate 180 degrees and mirror the image using your photo imaging software.

Again, give the patient a break while you prepare the next size mirror.

## Lateral Right Closed:
After warming the smaller mirror and drying it completely, tell the patient, "Place the left retractor in your mouth and turn your head to the right." Now place the mirror in the right side and tell the patient, "Close on all of your back teeth." Make sure you can see the plane of occlusion in the center of the mirror.

THE WAY OF THE SUPERIOR DENTIST

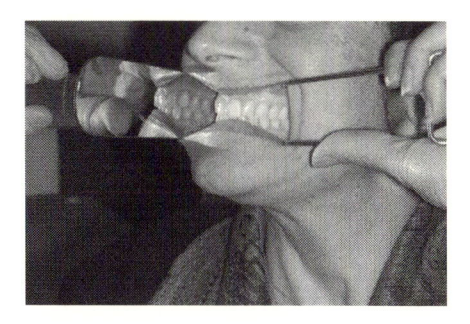

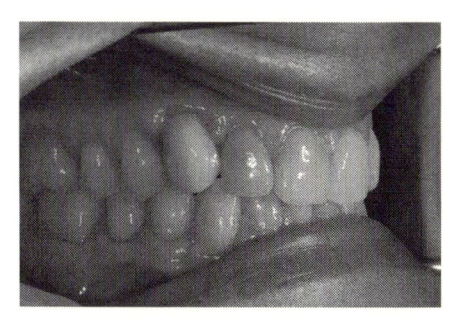

Note: After downloading this photo, in order to get the correct orientation, you must mirror the image using your photo imaging software.

### Lateral Right Open:
In the same exact position, ask the patient to open slightly until you can see the lower plane of occlusion.

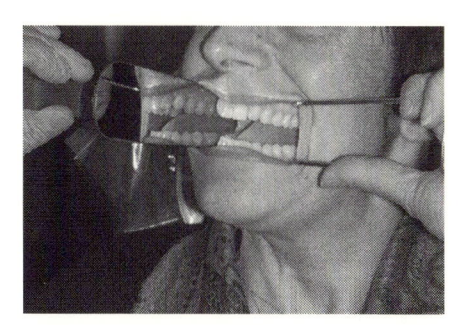

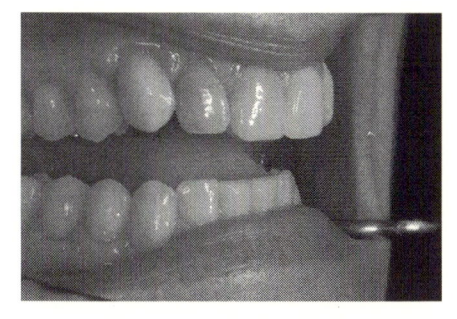

Note: After downloading this photo, in order to get the correct orientation, you must mirror the image using your photo imaging software.

### Lateral Left Closed:
When switching to the left side, stay on the patient's right side and ask the patient to place the retractor on the right side and look straight ahead. While

207

the patient's mouth remains open, place the mirror and tell him or her, "Bite down on all your back teeth."

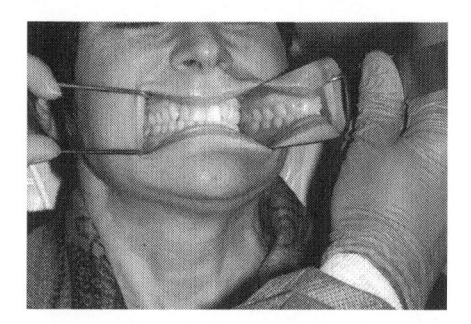

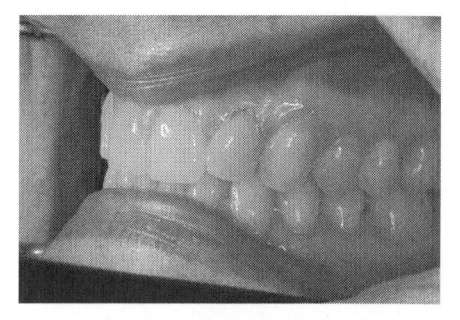

Note: After downloading this photo, in order to get the correct orientation, you must mirror the image using your photo imaging software.

Lateral Left Open:
Repeat the same process for the open position.

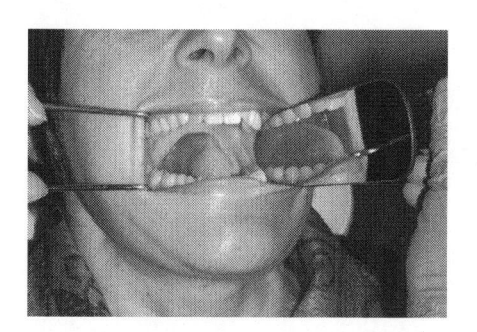

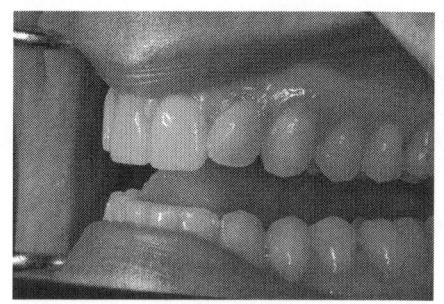

Note: After downloading this photo, in order to get the correct orientation, you must mirror the image using your photo imaging software.

## THE WAY OF THE SUPERIOR DENTIST

<u>**Portrait:**</u>
With a macro lens, you may find it difficult to step back far enough to get a reasonable portrait shot. To resolve this issue, have the patient stand against a wall that is far enough away to capture the entire head. Prior to taking the portrait shot, change the camera settings to the appropriate f-stop based on your particular camera system.

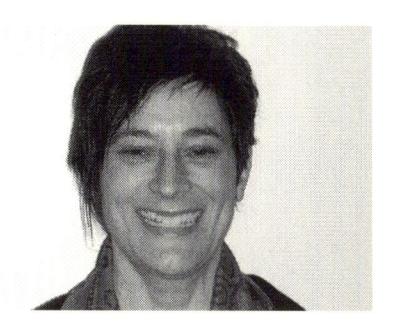

**APPENDIX 3**

# Image Used in Picture Exercise

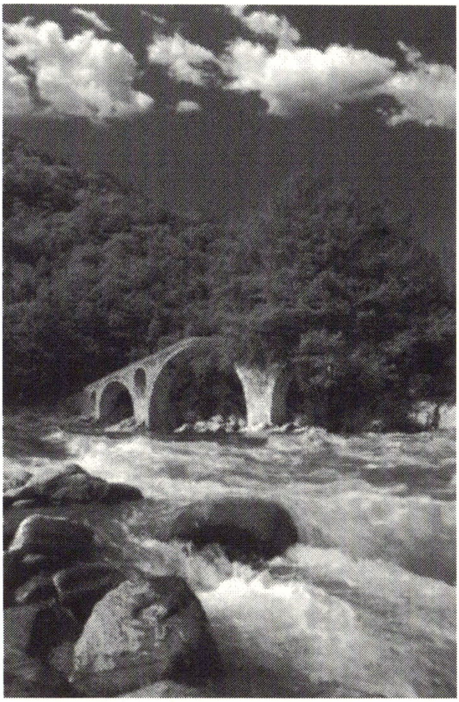

Figure 7: Picture from FreeDigitalPhotos.net.

# BIBLIOGRAPHY

Achor, S. *The Seven Principles of Positive Psychology That Fuel Success and Performance at Work.* New York: Crown Business, 2010.

Anonymous. (2007). *I go to the dentist today and am so scared?* Retrieved September 4, 2010, from Yahoo! Answers: http://answers.yahoo.com/question/index;_ylt=Alw4X.72QEn1dbwSEKztg_jrxQt.;_ylv=3?qid=20080118035043AAqOGa4

Chanpong, B. D., Haas, D. D., & Locker, D. D. "Need and Demand for Sedation or General Anesthesia in Dentistry: A National Survey of the Canadian Population," *Anesthesia Progress,* 52, (2005): 3–11.

Donaldson, M. R., Gizarelli, G. B., & Chanpong, B. D. "Oral Sedation: A Primer on Anxiolysis for the Adult Patient," *Anesthesia Progress,* 54 (2007): 118–29.

Hamer, R. D. (1990). *The Smith-Kettlewell Eye Research Institute.* Retrieved September 5, 2010, from What Can My Baby See?: http://www.ski.org/Vision/babyvision.html

Hanh, T. N. (2009, August 24). *Art of Mindful Living—Walking Meditation.* Retrieved August 12, 2010, from Plum Village: http://www.plumvillage.org/practice.html?start=28

Heath, C. A. *Made to Stick: Why Some Ideas Survive and Others Die.* New York: Random House, 2007.

Hutcherson, C. A., Seppala, E. M., & Gross, J. J. "Loving-Kindness Meditation Increases Social Connectedness," *Emotion, 8(5)* (2008): 720–4.

Smith, J. (2010, February 17). *Shamatha Project.* Retrieved August 12, 2010, from UC Davis Center for Mind and Brain: http://mindbrain.ucdavis.edu/people/jeremy/shamatha-project?searchterm=meditation+emotion.

Stalker, C. A., Carruthers, R., Teram, E., & Schachter, C. L. "Providing Dental Care to Survivors of Childhood Sexual Abuse: Treatment Considerations for the Practitioner," *The Journal of the American Dental Association, 136*(9) (2005): 1277–81.

*Taking the Bite Out.* (n.d.). Retrieved August 29, 2010, from MSNBC.Com: http://www.msnbc.msn.com/id/5446421/100604.

## ABOUT THE AUTHOR

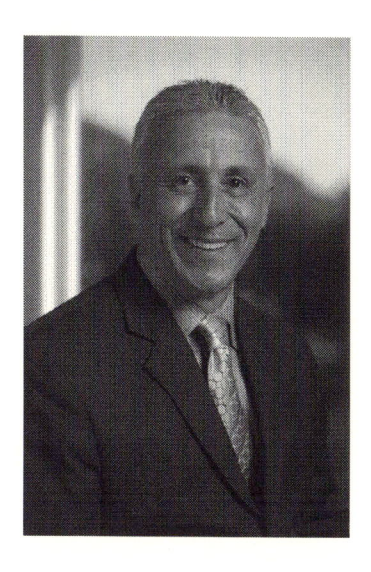

Adrian Wilkins is a dental consultant and coach to some of the country's premier dentists and dental practices. He is unique in his ability to motivate and coach dentists and teams to overcome limitations in their practices and lives. His services include individual coaching, dental consulting services, workshops, and motivational speaking, where he has presented nationally and internationally to audiences in excess of seven hundred dentists. His areas of expertise include leadership, personal development, case presentation for comprehensive care dentistry, branding, business strategy and systems, and dental practice organization.

Adrian is a partner in WHM Dental Consultants and has founded the nationwide marketing company Sedation Dentistry Network, LLC. He is a student and practitioner of organizational development, systems thinking, psychology, and communication. Adrian is also a certified master practitioner in neurolinguistics programming (NLP) and has been an adjunct professor at New York University.

Made in the USA
Charleston, SC
07 April 2014